Editors

ASIF M. ILYAS
SHITAL N. PARIKH
SAQIB REHMAN
GILES R. SCUDERI
FELASFA M. WODAJO

ORTHOPEDIC CLINICS
OF NORTH AMERICA

www.orthopedic.theclinics.com

January 2014 • Volume 45 • Number 1

ELSEVIER

1600 John F. Kennedy Boulevard • Suite 1800 • Philadelphia, Pennsylvania, 19103-2899.

http://www.orthopedic.theclinics.com

ORTHOPEDIC CLINICS OF NORTH AMERICA Volume 45, Number 1
January 2014 ISSN 0030-5898, ISBN-13: 978-0-323-26402-0

Editor: Jennifer Flynn-Briggs
Developmental Editor: Stephanie Carter

Orthopedic Clinics of North America (ISSN 0030-5898) is published quarterly by Elsevier Inc., 360 Park Avenue South, New York, NY 10010-1710. Months of issue are January, April, July, and October. Business and Editorial Offices: 1600 John F. Kennedy Blvd., Suite 1800, Philadelphia, PA 19103-2899. Customer Service Office: 3251 Riverport Lane, Maryland Heights, MO 63043. Periodicals postage paid at New York, NY and additional mailing offices. Subscription prices are $310.00 per year for (US individuals), $596.00 per year for (US institutions), $365.00 per year (Canadian individuals), $727.00 per year (Canadian institutions), $450.00 per year (international individuals), $727.00 per year (international institutions), $150.00 per year (US students), $220.00 per year (Canadian and international students). Foreign air speed delivery is included in all *Clinics* subscription prices. All prices are subject to change without notice. **POSTMASTER:** Send change of address to *Orthopedic Clinics of North America*, **Elsevier Health Sciences Division, Subscription Customer Service, 3251 Riverport Lane, Maryland Heights, MO 63043. Customer Service (orders, claims, online, change of address): Elsevier Health Sciences Division, Subscription Customer Service, 3251 Riverport Lane, Maryland Heights, MO 63043. Tel: 1-800-654-2452 (U.S. and Canada); 314-447-8871 (outside U.S. and Canada). Fax: 314-447-8029. E-mail: journalscustomerservice-usa@elsevier. com (for print support); journalsonlinesupport-usa@elsevier.com (for online support).**

Reprints. For copies of 100 or more, of articles in this publication, please contact the Commercial Reprints Department, Elsevier Inc., 360 Park Avenue South, New York, NY 10010-1710. Tel.: 212-633-3874; Fax: 212-633-3820; E-mail: reprints@elsevier. com.

Orthopedic Clinics of North America is covered in *MEDLINE/PubMed* (*Index Medicus*), *Cinahl, Excerpta Medica, and Cumulative Index to Nursing and Allied Health Literature.*

Printed in the United States of America.

Contributors

EDITORS

ASIF M. ILYAS, MD - *Upper Extremity*
Program Fellowship Director of Hand and
Upper Extremity Surgery, Rothman Institute,
Associate Professor of Orthopaedic Surgery,
Thomas Jefferson University, Philadelphia,
Pennsylvania

SHITAL N. PARIKH, MD - *Pediatrics*
Pediatric Orthopaedic Sports Medicine,
Associate Professor of Orthopaedic Surgery,
Cincinnati Children's Hospital Medical Center,
University of Cincinnati School of Medicine,
Cincinnati, Ohio

SAQIB REHMAN, MD - *Trauma*
Director of Orthopaedic Trauma, Associate
Professor of Orthopaedic Surgery, Temple
University Hospital, Philadelphia,
Pennsylvania

GILES R. SCUDERI, MD - *Adult
Reconstruction*
Vice President, Orthopedic Service Line,
Northshore LIJ Health System; Director, ISK
Institute, New York, New York

FELASFA M. WODAJO, MD - *Musculoskeletal
Oncology*
Musculoskeletal Tumor Surgery, Virginia
Hospital Center, Arlington, Virginia; Assistant
Professor, Orthopedic Surgery, Georgetown
University Hospital, Washington, DC; Assistant
Professor, Orthopedic Surgery, VCU School
of Medicine, Inova Campus, Falls Church,
Virginia

AUTHORS

JAIMO AHN, MD, PhD
Assistant Professor, Department of
Orthopaedic Surgery, Hospital of the University
of Pennsylvania, University of Pennsylvania,
Philadelphia, Pennsylvania

SANJEEV BHATIA, MD
Division of Sports Medicine, Department of
Orthopedic Surgery, Rush University Medical
Center, Rush Medical College of Rush
University, Chicago, Illinois

NICHOLAS CAGGIANO, MD
St. Luke's Orthopedic Specialists, Department
of Orthopaedic Surgery, St. Luke's University
Hospital, Bethlehem, Pennsylvania

PETER CHALMERS, MD
Division of Sports Medicine, Department of
Orthopedic Surgery, Rush University Medical
Center, Rush Medical College of Rush
University, Chicago, Illinois

FELIX H. CHEUNG, MD
Associate Professor and Vice Chair of
Operations and Finance, Chief, Orthopaedic
Oncology, Department of Orthopaedic
Surgery, Joan C Edwards School of Medicine,
Marshall University, Huntington, West Virginia

AKHIL CHHATRE, MD
Instructor, Department of Physical Medicine
and Rehabilitation; Instructor, Department of
Neurological Surgery, Johns Hopkins
University, Baltimore, Maryland

H. JOHN COOPER, MD
Assistant Medical Staff, Adult Reconstructive
Orthopaedic Surgery, Department of
Orthopaedic Surgery, Lenox Hill Hospital,
New York, New York

DANIELLE CROSS, MD
Department of Orthopaedic Surgery, St. Luke's
University Hospital, Bethlehem, Pennsylvania

CRAIG J. DELLA VALLE, MD
Director, Adult Joint Reconstruction
Fellowship, Rush University Medical Center,
Chicago, Illinois

DEREK DONEGAN, MD
Assistant Professor, Department of
Orthopaedic Surgery, Hospital of the University
of Pennsylvania, University of Pennsylvania,
Philadelphia, Pennsylvania

ANIL GUPTA, MD, MBA
Division of Sports Medicine, Department of
Orthopedic Surgery, Rush University Medical
Center, Rush Medical College of Rush
University, Chicago, Illinois

BRYAN D. HAUGHOM, MD
Orthopaedic Surgery Resident Physician, Rush
University Medical Center, Chicago, Illinois

JOSÉ HERRERA-SOTO, MD
Director of the Center for Orthopedics, Arnold
Palmer Hospital for Children, Orlando, Florida

ASHOT S. KOTCHARIAN, MD
PGY4 Resident Physician, Department of
Physical Medicine and Rehabilitation,
University of Pennsylvania Perelman School of
Medicine, Philadelphia, Pennsylvania

KRISTOFER S. MATULLO, MD
Head of the Division of Hand Surgery, Chief of
Hand Surgery, Department of Orthopaedic
Surgery, St. Luke's University Hospital and
Health Network, Bethlehem; Assistant Clinical
Professor of Orthopaedic Surgery, Temple
University Hospital, Philadelphia, Pennsylvania

FRANK MCCORMICK, MD
Midwest Orthopaedics at Rush, Rush
University Medical Center, Chicago, Illinois

SAMIR MEHTA, MD
Assistant Professor, Chief, Division of
Orthopaedic Trauma, Department of
Orthopaedic Surgery, Hospital of the University
of Pennsylvania, University of Pennsylvania,
Philadelphia, Pennsylvania

HASSAN MIR, MD
Assistant Professor, Division of Orthopaedic
Trauma, Vanderbilt Orthopaedic Institute,
Vanderbilt Medical Center, Nashville,
Tennessee

RONAK M. PATEL, MD
Chief Resident, Department of Orthopaedic
Surgery, Feinberg School of Medicine,
Northwestern University, Chicago, Illinois

KATHRYN PECK, MD
Hand and Upper Extremity Fellow, The Indiana
Hand to Shoulder Center, Indianapolis,
Indianapolis

CHRISTOPHER T. PLASTARAS, MD
Assistant Professor, Department of Physical
Medicine and Rehabilitation, University of
Pennsylvania Perelman School of Medicine,
Philadelphia, Pennsylvania

DARREN R. PLUMMER, MBA
Adult Joint Reconstructive Clinical Research
Fellow, Department of Orthopaedic Surgery,
Rush University Medical Center, Chicago,
Illinois

ANTHONY A. ROMEO, MD
Division of Sports Medicine, Department of
Orthopedic Surgery, Rush University Medical
Center, Rush Medical College of Rush
University, Chicago, Illinois

JAMES M. SCHUSTER, MD, PhD
Associate Professor, Department of
Neurological Surgery, Hospital of the University
of Pennsylvania, Philadelphia, Pennsylvania

**HITESH SHAH, MS (Orthopaedics), DNB
(Orthopaedics)**
Associate Professor, Pediatric Orthopaedic
Services, Department of Orthopaedics,
Kasturba Medical College, Manipal University,
Manipal, Karnataka, India

HERRICK J. SIEGEL, MD
Professor of Surgery, Section Head,
Orthopaedic Oncology, University of Alabama
at Birmingham Medical Center, Birmingham,
Alabama

HARVEY E. SMITH, MD
Assistant Professor, Department of
Orthopaedic Surgery, Pennsylvania Hospital,
University of Pennsylvania, Philadelphia,
Pennsylvania

DANIEL J. STINNER, MD
Fellow, Orthopaedic Trauma, Division of
Orthopaedic Trauma, Vanderbilt Orthopaedic
Institute, Vanderbilt Medical Center, Nashville,
Tennessee

S. DAVID STULBERG, MD
Clinical Professor of Orthopaedic Surgery,
Department of Orthopaedic Surgery, Feinberg
School of Medicine, Northwestern University,
Chicago, Illinois

MATTHEW P. SULLIVAN, MD
Resident, Department of Orthopaedic Surgery,
Hospital of the University of Pennsylvania,
University of Pennsylvania, Philadelphia,
Pennsylvania

NIKHIL VERMA, MD
Division of Sports Medicine, Department of
Orthopedic Surgery, Rush University Medical
Center, Rush Medical College of Rush
University, Chicago, Illinois

Contents

encountered apex anterior and/or valgus deformities remains a challenge when treating these injuries. It is necessary for the surgeon to recognize this and know how to neutralize these forces. Surgeons should be comfortable using a variety of the reduction techniques presented to minimize fracture malalignment.

Peripheral nerve traction injuries may occur after surgical care and can involve any of the upper extremity large peripheral nerves. In this review, injuries after shoulder or elbow surgical intervention are discussed. Understanding the varying mechanisms of injury as well as classification is imperative for preoperative risk stratification as well as management.

Peripheral nerve traction injuries may occur after surgical care and can involve any of the lower extremity large peripheral nerves. In this review, the authors discuss injuries after knee or hip surgical intervention. The diagnosis, including electrodiagnostic studies, is time sensitive and also relies on a detailed history and physical examination. Successful prevention and treatment involve familiarity with risk and predisposing factors as well as prophylactic measures.

Spondylopelvic dissociation is a complex injury pattern resulting in multiplanar instability of the lumbopelvis. These injuries have traditionally been known as "suicide jumper's fractures" and have recently increased in prevalence as a result of under-vehicle explosions seen in the past decade of military conflicts in the Middle East. The hallmarks of spondylopelvic dissociation are bilateral vertical sacral fractures with a horizontal component, resulting in lumbosacral instability in the sagittal and axial planes. Surgical treatment has evolved greatly and both percutaneous and open options are available, with triangular osteosynthesis being the most relied on method of fixation.

Pediatrics

Slipped capital femoral epiphysis (SCFE) is a common hip disorder among adolescents, whereby the epiphysis is displaced posteriorly and inferiorly to the metaphysis. Treatment modalities aim to stabilize the epiphysis, prevent further slippage, and avoid complications associated with long-term morbidity, such as osteonecrosis and chondrolysis. Controversy exists with SCFE regarding prophylactic fixation of the contralateral, painless, normal hip, the role of femoroacetabular impingement with SCFE, and whether in situ fixation is the best treatment method for SCFE. This article presents and discusses the latest diagnostic and treatment modalities for SCFE.

Perthes disease refers to self-limiting idiopathic avascular necrosis of capital femoral epiphysis in a child. There is no consensus for the optimum treatment of Perthes disease even 100 years after the first description. The prime aim of the treatment is to maintain the sphericity of the femoral head and the congruency of the femur-acetabulum relationship to prevent secondary degenerative arthritis. Early diagnosis and management can help the collapse of femoral head, progressive femoral head deformity, and impingement.

Oncology

The management of complex wounds remains a challenge, and although there have been many promising advances, patients often undergo a morbid and lengthy process to obtain sufficient, satisfactory healing. Sarcoma patients are especially vulnerable to soft tissue wound-healing complications. These patients are often treated with neoadjuvant radiation and/or chemotherapy and have compromised local vascularity to healing tissue. The advent and refinement of wound vacuum-assisted closure technology have been shown to have a tremendous impact. This article reviews the benefits of some novel technologies currently undergoing investigation in orthopedic oncology that will likely have applications in wound management from other causes.

Long bone skeletal metastases are common in the United States, with more than 280,000 new cases every year. Most of these will be managed by the on-call orthopedic surgeon. A practical primer is offered for the evaluation and surgical management for the practicing orthopedist, including questions to ask during the history, pertinent physical examination findings, appropriate imaging requests, proper laboratory work, and biopsy options. Finally, 7 scenarios are presented to encompass most situations a practicing orthopedic surgeon will encounter, and guidelines for treatment and referral are offered.

Upper Extremity

Arthroscopic repair of type II superior labral anterior to posterior (SLAP) tears is currently the standard of care, with most patients obtaining good to excellent surgical results. However, overhead athletes and older patients have inferior outcomes.

Recent clinical studies and biomechanical data suggest that a biceps tenodesis is a suitable alternative in select patients. This article reviews the literature to identify the biomechanical and clinical indications for performing a biceps tenodesis for type II SLAP lesions.

The scaphoid is stabilized by the scapholunate ligament (directly) and lunotriquetral ligament (indirectly). Disruption of either of these ligaments leads to a pattern of instability that, left untreated, leads to altered mechanics of the wrist and ultimately debilitating arthritis and collapse. Although arthroscopy remains the gold standard for diagnosis of these injuries, plain films and advanced imaging are useful adjuncts. In the acute setting, conservative treatment may be attempted, but recalcitrant cases require surgical stabilization. Salvage procedures are also available for those patients who fail initial stabilization or present with late degeneration.

Kienböck disease, or osteonecrosis of the lunate, most often affects patients between the ages of 20 and 40 years. There are 4 major stages of the disease, and treatment is based on the stage of disease. Advancements are still being made with regards to the cause, pathophysiology, and preferred method of treatment of each stage. Although the goals of pain relief, motion preservation, strength maintenance, and function outcomes are paramount to success, no 1 procedure consistently and reliably achieves these outcomes. Further advancements in treatment and results of long-term outcome studies should resolve some of these topics.

ORTHOPEDIC CLINICS OF NORTH AMERICA

FORTHCOMING ISSUES

Beginning with the July 2013 issue, *Orthopedic Clinics of North America* will appear in this new format. Rather than focusing on a single topic, each issue will contain articles on key areas in orthopedics—adult reconstruction, upper extremity, trauma, pediatric and oncology. Articles on sports medicine and foot and ankle will also be included on a regular basis. As the practice of orthopedics has become more specialized, the format of one topic per issue is no longer fulfilling our readers' needs. The new format is intended to address these changing needs.

Orthopedic Clinics of North America will continue to publish a print issue four times a year, in January, April, July, and October. However, it will also include online-only articles that will be published on a rolling basis (not in accordance with our quarterly publication dates). These articles, along with articles from our print issues, will be available on http://www.orthopedic.theclinics.com/.

RECENT ISSUES

April 2013
Osteoporosis and Fragility Fractures
Jason A. Lowe, and Gary E. Friedlaender, *Editors*

January 2013
Emerging Concepts in Upper Extremity Trauma
Michael P. Leslie, and Seth D. Dodds, *Editors*

YOUR iPhone and iPad

Adult Reconstruction

Preface
Adult Reconstruction

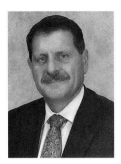

Giles R. Scuderi, MD
Editor

Total hip arthroplasty is one of the most common and successful procedures in orthopedics. With its popularity, numerous prosthetic options and approaches have been employed. The introduction of modular components, femoral components of various shapes, and alternative articulations has made it easier to reconstruct the arthritic hip joint. The intention is to preserve bone stock, while inserting a stable implant through various limited or extensile approaches. Modular components have made the procedure more adaptable to surgical variation, but have introduced the potential complication of metal corrosion at the head-neck interface or neck-body interface with the release of metal debris, resulting in a spectrum of effects such as adverse local tissue reaction, component failure, instability, or osteolysis. Dual mobility bearing hip designs are an alternative to standard articulations with greater stability and may serve as an alternative to large-diameter heads and constrained liners. Uncemented femoral components are designed in various shapes to address the broad spectrum of proximal femoral morphology. Some design features are advantageous, while others have potential consequences.

This issue focuses on several current topics that are relevant to modern hip arthroplasty, including metal corrosion with modular components, dual mobility bearing hip designs, and short uncemented stems.

Giles R. Scuderi, MD
Orthopedic Service Line
Northshore LIJ Health System
New York, NY, USA

ISK Institute
New York, NY, USA

E-mail address:
gscuderi@nshs.edu

orthopedic.theclinics.com

Dual Mobility in Total Hip Arthroplasty

Darren R. Plummer, MBA, Bryan D. Haughom, MD,
Craig J. Della Valle, MD*

KEYWORDS

- Dual-mobility • Total hip arthroplasty • Revision total hip arthroplasty • Dislocation

KEY POINTS

- Instability continues to be among the most common complications and reasons for revision of a total hip arthroplasty (THA) in North America.
- There is increasing interest in dual-mobility bearings as an alternative to standard articulations, as they are associated with a low risk of instability following both primary and revision THA and may serve as an alternative to traditional solutions for instability including large diameter heads and constrained liners.
- The 2 primary concerns with dual-mobility cups remain wear and intraprosthetic dislocation (IPD).
- IPD is a unique complication reported with dual-mobility implants, and further research is essential to clearly delineate the underlying mechanism of failure to adequately address this complication.
- Concern for increased wear over time and limited data on long-term survivorship in younger patients are concerns as the usage of these implants increases in North America.

INTRODUCTION

Total hip arthroplasty (THA) is one of the most successful and cost-effective procedures in orthopedics.[1,2] It effectively treats pain, improves function, and improves quality of life in patients with end-stage arthritis of the hip.[3] Instability, however, remains a persistent problem, and both the most common cause for revision of a THA and one of the most common complications seen postoperatively resulting in patient morbidity as well as substantial expense.[4] Numerous prosthetic options and surgical approaches have been attempted to both prevent and treat instability, including alternative approaches to the hip, capsular repair, larger femoral heads, and in some cases constrained liners. By virtue of their dual articulation, large jump distance and greater range of motion until impingement occurs, dual-mobility articulations are an attractive option to both prevent and treat instability.

HISTORY OF DUAL MOBILITY

Although dual-mobility articulations are relatively new to the US market, variations on the concept have been used clinically in Europe for more than 35 years. Bousquet developed the first model in the early 1970s in an effort to reduce the incidence of dislocations following primary THA. His development of the dual-mobility articulation is thought to blend the advantages of several attractive

Disclosures: The authors have not received any financial support for the work. Dr C.J. Della Valle is a consultant for Biomet, Convatec, Depuy, and Smith-& Nephew. He receives research support from Biomet, CD Diagnostics, Smith & Nephew, and Stryker. He is on the scientific advisory board for CD Diagnostics and owns stock and options in the company.
Department of Orthopaedic Surgery, Rush University Medical Center, 1611 West Harrison Street, Suite 300, Chicago, IL 60612, USA
* Corresponding author.
E-mail address: craigdv@yahoo.com

Orthop Clin N Am 45 (2014) 1–8
http://dx.doi.org/10.1016/j.ocl.2013.08.004

design options. Not only did the original dual-mobility design take advantage of the inherent stability imparted by a larger femoral head as originally proposed by McKee,[4] it also utilized the low-friction arthroplasty concept as described by John Charnley.[5] Bousquet's dual-mobility design incorporated a cementless metallic acetabular shell and a mobile polyethylene liner component that positively captured a larger prosthetic femoral head, allowing for greater range of motion within the socket and a low risk of dislocation when used for primary and revision THA as well as in the treatment of femoral neck fractures, a patient subset that is notorious for a high risk of instability.[6]

The evolution of Bousquet's innovative design has led to numerous modifications, including those aimed to improve cup fixation, decrease polyethylene wear, and decrease the rates of intra-prosthetic and complete dislocation, including alterations to the fixation surfaces and both the cup configuration and mating femoral neck design. First-generation dual-mobility cups relied upon press-fit fixation consisting of 2 pegs that were driven into the pubis and ischium, as well as a screw in the dome combined with an alumina coating sintered onto a nonporous surface. The result of this design resulted in high rates of delamination, third body wear, and loosening.[7,8] Subsequent generations of the dual mobility design no longer utilize an alumina coating, but rather use a dual layer coating of hydroxyapatite and titanium plasma spray to create a more 3-dimensional surface for osseointegration. Additionally, modifications have included changing the shape of the cup to decrease anterior overhang, which may both improve press-fit fixation and prevent iliopsoas tendon irritation.[9] Modifications to the femoral neck have focused on decreasing impingement around the introitus of the mobile polyethylene insert via a highly polished surface and a thin femoral neck. In general, the use of skirted femoral heads is also avoided in an effort to prevent impingement and subsequent intraprosthetic dislocation (IPD). Modifications to the liner have included the introduction of highly cross-linked polyethylene in an effort to decrease wear.[10,11] These modifications and design innovations have effectively resulted in decreased dislocation rates and improved cup survival. The survivorship rates published suggest little or no excess wear associated with dual-mobility implants.[6,12–14]

BIOMECHANICS OF DUAL MOBILITY

Dual-mobility designs incorporate 2 distinct articulations: the first between the femoral head and the polyethylene liner, and the second at the interface between the convex surface of the polyethylene liner and the acetabular shell. The primary articulation is between the femoral head and the polyethylene liner and is engaged during the majority of activities with normal range-of-motion requirements. The secondary articulation, between the polyethylene liner and the acetabular shell, is engaged during activities that exceed normal range of motion, when the neck of the femoral stem contacts the rim of the liner. These 2 articulations allow for greater range of motion, a greater head-to-neck ratio, and a more physiologic effective head size that increases the jump distance and hence resistance to dislocation. Laboratory studies have shown increased range of motion with dual-mobility versus traditional implants. Additionally, a greater distance-to-impingement imparted by the dual articulations has been correlated with decreased impingement and subsequent dislocations.[15,16] Guyen and colleagues[15] experimentally evaluated the range of motion to impingement of dual-mobility implants with 22.2 mm and 28 mm femoral head sizes. The authors found increased range of motion with the dual-mobility implants compared with standard implants, reporting increased flexion of 30.5°, adduction of 15.4°, and external rotation of 22.4° in the dual-mobility implants.[15]

NORTH AMERICAN EXPERIENCE

Only recently has the use of dual-mobility components gained popularity in the United States, with several designs now commercially available following the US Food and Drug Administration (FDA) approval of the first design in 2009. Although several of these designs are ones that have prior experience in Europe, newer designs for the US market include acetabular components with cobalt alloy counter bearings (as opposed to stainless steel as is used widely in Europe), titanium fixation surfaces, and cross-linked polyethylenes.

The Active Articulation E1 dual-mobility hip system (Biomet, Warsaw, Indiana) (**Fig. 1**) includes a cementless cup with a high carbon cobalt chrome molybdenum alloy bearing surface and titanium porous plasma spray coating. The polyethylene liner is highly cross-linked and infused with vitamin E, which potentially prevents oxidative degeneration and increases strength.[17] Although simulated wear studies conducted by the manufacturer suggest a significant reduction in polyethylene wear is achieved with the vitamin E-infused polyethylene, bearing retrieval analysis and clinical studies are still necessary to validate these claims.

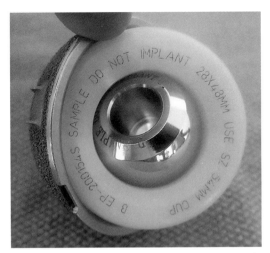

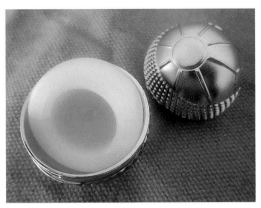

Fig. 2. POLARCUP dual-mobility hip system by Smith & Nephew Orthopedics, which is available in versions for cementless (*left*) and cemented (*right*) use.

Fig. 1. Active Articulation E1 dual-mobility system by Biomet Orthopedics.

The POLARCUP dual-mobility hip system (Smith & Nephew, Memphis, Tennessee) (**Fig. 2**) has a more than 10-year history of clinical use in Europe and has been more recently released in the United States with both cementless and cemented versions. Specific design features include a liner that limits contact between the liner and the neck of the femoral stem. This implant includes a stainless steel bearing surface and a titanium plasma spray fixation surface. A retrospective analysis of 150 primary THAs using the POLARCUP dual-mobility hip showed a 97.4% survivorship at 7.1 years using aseptic loosening as a primary end point, with no dislocations reported.[14]

Stryker Orthopaedics (Mahwah, New Jersey) offers 2 dual-mobility systems, the Restoration Anatomic Dual-Mobility (ADM) and Modular Dual-Mobility (MDM) X3 Mobile Bearing Acetabular systems (**Fig. 3**). The ADM implant is a monoblock shell with a cobalt alloy bearing surface and a titanium plasma spray fixation surface that is coated with hydroxyapatite. It is anatomically designed (requiring right and left implants) with a psoas tendon cutout potentially reducing tendon impingement. The MDM design is unique in that it has a modular cobalt alloy liner, which engages into a more standard acetabular component, which allows for adjunctive screw fixation. Although the ADM offers a 6 mm nominal size difference between the head and shell, the MDM head-to-cup difference is 12 mm; the use of adjunctive screw fixation, however, lends itself more to use in the setting of revision procedures.

DUAL MOBILITY IN PRIMARY THA

The dual-mobility socket was originally designed to be used in patients undergoing primary THA who were considered to be at high risk for dislocation. Current literature suggests those patients

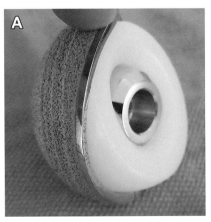

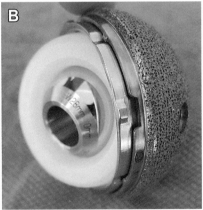

Fig. 3. (*A*) Restoration Anatomic Dual-Mobility (ADM) X3 dual-mobility hip system by Stryker Orthopaedics. (*B*) Modular Dual-mobility (MDM) X3 dual-mobility hip system by Stryker Orthopaedics.

Table 1
Dual mobility in primary THA

Author, Year	Number of Hips	Mean Patient Age in Years (Range)	Mean Follow-up in Years (Range)	Dislocation Rate (%)	Revision Rate	Cup Design	Survivorship of Cup
Phillippot et al,[6] 2009	384	55.8 (23–87)	15.3 (12–20)	3.6	8.9% (34 out of 384); 13 aseptic loosening, 14 IPD, 7 liner exchanges for wear	Novae-1 titanium; Novae-1 stainless steel (SERF)	96.7% @ 15 y
Bauchu et al,[14] 2008	150	69 (40.3–90.5)	6.2 (3.3–7.1)	0	1.3% (2 out of 150) revised for aseptic loosening	3rd generation POLARCUP (Smith & Nephew)	97.4% @ 7.1 y
Bouchet et al,[25] 2011	105	75 (70–81)	2.3 (1.2–3.6)	0	Not reported	Novae; Stafit; Avantage; Gyros cups	Not reported
Farizon et al,[13] 1998	135	63 (27–89)	6.4 (0–11.8)	0.7	3.7% (5 out of 135) 4 revised for aseptic loosening; 1 dislocation	Novae-1 cup (SERF)	95.4% @ 12 y
Hamadouche et al,[23] 2012	168	67 (18–92)	6 (5–8)	2	2% (4 out of 168); 4 IPD	Tregor unconstrained tripolar cup (Aston Medical)	94.2% @ 7 y
Guyen et al,[22] 2007	167	72 (21–97)	3.4 (2–5.4)	0	3.6% (6 out of 167); 2 deep infections, 1 aseptic loosening, 1 periprosthetic femur fracture, 1 post-traumatic acetabular discontinuity, 1 trochanteric nonunion	Saturne cup (Amplitude)	96.4% @ 5 y
Boyer et al,[12] 2012	240	55 (30–70)	22	0	17.2% (42 out of 240); 20 for aseptic loosening, 2 for septic loosening, 10 for IPD, 5 for liner wear, 5 for loose stem	Novae tripodal (SERF)	80% @ 22 y

at high risk of dislocation include patients older than 75 years; patients with a history of prior hip surgery, neuromuscular disease, higher Charlson comorbidity or American Society of Anesthesiologists score; and patients undergoing primary THA for a femoral neck fracture.[18–20] Multiple studies have shown decreased instability and lower dislocation rates in primary THA with dual-mobility implants, resulting in the use of dual mobility implants for primary THA in younger, lower-risk patients or as a treatment method for recurrent instability.[8,12,21–24] Studies report dislocation rates of dual-mobility implants ranging from 0% to 3.6% in primary THAs (**Table 1**).[6,12–14,22,23,25] Most published studies evaluate an older patient population (>65 years), with limited data on younger, more active patients, and care should be taken when using dual-mobility bearings in this patient demographic, in whom wear could become more problematic.

The dual-mobility concept is not without problems and potential concerns, however, and other than failures of fixation (which may have been related to suboptimal fixation surfaces), complications related to the polyethylene bearing are a concern. Specifically, dual-mobility implants not only have thinner polyethylene liners, but potentially accelerated wear imparted by the 2 articulating surfaces. There is further concern over potential higher wear rates on the convex surface of a polyethylene bearing. Wear around the introitus of the bearing, as previously described, can lead to IPD of the bearing, most frequently reported in younger patients at an average of 6 to 8 years postoperatively secondary to polyethylene liner wear.[9,21,23]

IPD is a specific complication encountered with dual-mobility articulations, induced by loss of the polyethylene retentive rim resulting in separation of the femoral head from the polyethylene liner. Some of the reported implant-related factors associated with IPD include large-diameter femoral necks, smaller head-to-neck ratios, and longer neck lengths that include a skirt.[23,26] Rates of IPD vary based on implant design, from 1.9% to 5.2% reported with older-generation dual-mobility designs at a mean follow-up of 4 to 17 years[8,9,27] and from 0% to 2.4% with more current dual-mobility designs at follow-up periods ranging from 6 to 9 years (**Table 2**).[7,21,23,28]

DUAL MOBILITY IN REVISION THA

The risk of recurrent dislocation is greater after revision surgery than primary THA,[19,29–31] and hence the use of dual mobility is attractive for revision procedures and for the treatment of the hip that is unstable, as an alternative to conventional larger-diameter (>36 mm) femoral heads and constrained liners. Overall, dislocation rates using dual mobility

Table 2
IPD in dual mobility

Author, Year	Number of Hips	Average Patient Age in Years (Range)	Follow-up Period Average in Years (Range)	IPD Rate (%)	Cup Design
Combes et al,[21] 2013	2480	69 (19–94)	7 (0.17–11)	0.28	Multiple cup designs[a]
Hamadouche et al,[23] 2012	168	67 (18–92)	6 (5–8)	2.0	Tregor unconstrained tripolar cup (Aston Medical)
Vielpeau et al,[28] 2011	668	67.5 (25–92)	9 (5–16)	0.69[a] 0[b]	[a]Original Bousquet design; Novae-E cup (SERF)
Massin et al,[7] 2012	2601	72 (55–92)	7.7 (5–11)	0.12	Multiple cup designs (all 2nd generation designs)
Philippot et al,[8] 2008	438	54.8 (23–87)	17 (12–20)	5.3	Novae-1 titanium cups and Novae-1 stainless steel cups (SERF)
Philippot et al,[9] 2013	1960	51 (21–85)	14 (11–25)	4	Novae-1 cups (SERF)
Guyen et al,[27] 2009	54	66.5 (36–99)	4 (2.2–6.8)	3.7	Saturne cup (Amplitude)

[a] All patients received hemispherical dual-mobility cups. The study did not specify with which cups IPDs occurred;
[b] Novae-E cup (SERF).

Table 3
Dual mobility in revision THA

Author, Year	Number of Hips	Mean Patient Age in Years (Range)	Mean Follow-up in Years (Range)	Dislocation Rate (%)	Revision Rate	Cup Design	Survivorship of Cup
Hamadouche et al,[40] 2010	51	71 (41.1–91.8)	4.3 (2.1–6.4)	4.3	2% (1 out of 51) for acetabular component loosening	Medial cup (Aston Medical)	96% @ 6 y
Leiber-Wackenheim et al,[32] 2011	59	68 (47–88)	8 (6–11)	1.7	6.8% (4 out of 59); 1 dislocation, 1 femoral fracture, 1 infection, 1 hematoma	Novae-1; Novae-E (SERF)	98% @ 8 y
Guyen et al,[27] 2009	54	67 (35.7–98.7)	3.9 (2.2–6.8)	5.5	9.2% (5 out of 54); 2 dislocations, 3 deep infections	Saturne cup (Amplitude)	90.8% @ 6 y
Philippot et al,[30] 2009	163	68.7 (34–92)	5 (3.6–6.5)	3.7	6.7% (11 out of 163); 2 periprosthetic fractures, 3 deep infections, 2 trochanter nonunion, 1 femoral implant fracture, 2 aseptic loosening, 1 PE liner exchange for wear	Novae series (SERF); Sunfit; Stick; Novae-1; Coptos	96.1% @ 7 y
Hailer et al,[41] 2012	228	93 patient 60–75; 115>75	2 (0–6)	2	8.0% (18 out of 228); 5 for deep infection, 4 dislocation, 4 aseptic loosening, 3 for fracture, 2 other	Avantage cup	93% @ 2 y
Langlais et al,[42] 2008	85	72 (65–86)	3.5 (2–5)	1.1	8.0% (6 out of 85); 1 dislocation, 2 for deep infections, 3 for traumatic fracture below stem	Medial cup (Aston Medical)	94.6% @ 5 y

in revision THA[27,32,33] appear to be lower than those reported in revision THA with conventional implants. Further, several studies have examined the use of dual mobility specifically for the treatment of recurrent instability. Short- to midterm studies (2–11 years) have demonstrated excellent outcomes with regards to low rates of aseptic loosening and dislocation (**Table 3**).[27,30,34,35]

DUAL MOBILITY IN FEMORAL NECK FRACTURES

Although THA has been shown to be associated with excellent clinical outcomes and a lower risk of revision that hemiarthroplasty for the treatment of displaced femoral neck fractures in ambulatory patients, high dislocation rates have been reported consistently.[34–39] Recent meta-analyses found dislocation rates ranging from 9% to 10.7% in patients with femoral neck fractures treated with THA.[34,35] A recent study by Tarasevicius and colleagues[37] compared dual-mobility implants with conventional THA (performed with 28 mm and 32 mm femoral heads through a posterior approach) for the treatment of FNF. At 1 year postoperative follow-up, no dislocations were reported in the dual-mobility group compared with 8 (14.3%) dislocations in the conventional THA group.[37] In a similar study, Adam and colleagues[38] reported 3 (1.4%) dislocations at 9 month follow-up in 214 patients treated with dual-mobility implants for FNFs. The low dislocation rates reported in these studies support the consideration of dual-mobility implants to treat FNFs in elderly patients.

SUMMARY

Instability continues to be among the most common complications and reasons for revision of a THA in North America. Hence there is increasing interest in dual-mobility bearings as an alternative to standard articulations, as they are associated with a low risk of instability following primary and revision THA. Additionally, they may serve as an alternative to traditional solutions for instability including large-diameter heads and constrained liners. The 2 primary concerns with dual-mobility cups remain wear and IPD. IPD is a unique complication reported with dual-mobility implants, and further research is essential to clearly delineate the underlying mechanism of failure to adequately address this complication. Furthermore, concern for increased wear over time and limited data on long-term survivorship in younger patients are concerns as the usage of these implants increases in North America.

REFERENCES

1. Austin MS, Higuera CA, Rothman RH. Total hip arthroplasty at the Rothman Institute. HSS J 2012; 8(2):146–50.
2. NIH consensus conference: total hip replacement. NIH Consensus Development Panel on Total Hip Replacement. JAMA 1995;273(24):1950–6.
3. Huo MH, Parvizi J, Bal BS, et al. What's new in total hip arthroplasty. J Bone Joint Surg Am 2009;91(10): 2522–34.
4. Bozic KJ, Kurtz SM, Lau E, et al. The epidemiology of revision total hip arthroplasty in the United States. J Bone Joint Surg Am 2009;91(1):128–33.
5. Waugh W. John Charnley: the man and the hip. London, New York: Springer Verlag; 1990.
6. Philippot R, Camilleri JP, Boyer B, et al. The use of a dual-articulation acetabular cup system to prevent dislocation after primary total hip arthroplasty: analysis of 384 cases at a mean follow-up of 15 years. Int Orthop 2009;33(4):927–32.
7. Massin P, Orain V, Philippot R, et al. Fixation failures of dual mobility cups: a mid-term study of 2601 hip replacements. Clin Orthop Relat Res 2012;470(7): 1932–40.
8. Philippot R, Farizon F, Camilleri JP, et al. Survival of cementless dual mobility socket with a mean 17 years follow-up. Rev Chir Orthop Reparatrice Appar Mot 2008;94(8):e23–7.
9. Philippot R, Boyer B, Farizon F. Intraprosthetic dislocation: a specific complication of the dual-mobility system. Clin Orthop Relat Res 2013;471(3):965–70.
10. Galvin A, Kang L, Tipper J, et al. Wear of crosslinked polyethylene under different tribological conditions. J Mater Sci Mater Med 2006;17(3):235–43.
11. Glyn-Jones S, Isaac S, Hauptfleisch J, et al. Does highly cross-linked polyethylene wear less than conventional polyethylene in total hip arthroplasty? A double-blind, randomized, and controlled trial using roentgen stereophotogrammetric analysis. J Arthroplasty 2008;23(3):337–43.
12. Boyer B, Philippot R, Geringer J, et al. Primary total hip arthroplasty with dual mobility socket to prevent dislocation: a 22-year follow-up of 240 hips. Int Orthop 2012;36(3):511–8.
13. Farizon F, de Lavison R, Azoulai JJ, et al. Results with a cementless alumina-coated cup with dual mobility. A twelve-year follow-up study. Int Orthop 1998;22(4):219–24.
14. Bauchu P, Bonnard O, Cypres A, et al. The dual-mobility POLARCUP: first results from a multicenter study. Orthopedics 2008;31(12 Suppl 2):97–9.
15. Guyen O, Chen QS, Bejui-Hugues J, et al. Unconstrained tripolar hip implants: effect on hip stability. Clin Orthop Relat Res 2007;455:202–8.
16. Ghaffari M, Nickmanesh R, Tamannaee N, et al. The impingement-dislocation risk of total hip

replacement: effects of cup orientation and patient maneuvers. Conf Proc IEEE Eng Med Biol Soc 2012;2012:6801–4.

17. Greene MB, Freiberg C, Kwon A, et al. RSA Evaluation of wear of vitamin E stabilized highly cross-linked polyethylene. Paper No. 15. AAKS. 2010.

18. Jolles BM, Zangger P, Leyvraz PF. Factors predisposing to dislocation after primary total hip arthroplasty: a multivariate analysis. J Arthroplasty 2002; 17(3):282–8.

19. Alberton GM, High WA, Morrey BF. Dislocation after revision total hip arthroplasty: an analysis of risk factors and treatment options. J Bone Joint Surg Am 2002;84(10):1788–92.

20. Prokopetz JJ, Losina E, Bliss RL, et al. Risk factors for revision of primary total hip arthroplasty: a systematic review. BMC Musculoskelet Disord 2012; 13:251.

21. Combes A, Migaud H, Girard J, et al. Low rate of dislocation of dual-mobility cups in primary total hip arthroplasty. Clin Orthop Relat Res 2013. [Epub ahead of print].

22. Guyen O, Pibarot V, Vaz G, et al. Unconstrained tripolar implants for primary total hip arthroplasty in patients at risk for dislocation. J Arthroplasty 2007; 22(6):849–58.

23. Hamadouche M, Arnould H, Bouxin B. Is a cementless dual mobility socket in primary THA a reasonable option? Clin Orthop Relat Res 2012;470(11): 3048–53.

24. Philippot R, Adam P, Farizon F, et al. Survival of cementless dual mobility sockets: ten-year follow-up. Rev Chir Orthop Reparatrice Appar Mot 2006; 92(4):326–31.

25. Bouchet R, Mercier N, Saragaglia D. Posterior approach and dislocation rate: a 213 total hip replacements case-control study comparing the dual mobility cup with a conventional 28-mm metal head/polyethylene prosthesis. Orthop Traumatol Surg Res 2011;97(1):2–7.

26. Lecuire F, Benareau I, Rubini J, et al. Intra-prosthetic dislocation of the Bousquet dual mobility socket. Rev Chir Orthop Reparatrice Appar Mot 2004; 90(3):249–55.

27. Guyen O, Pibarot V, Vaz G, et al. Use of a dual mobility socket to manage total hip arthroplasty instability. Clin Orthop Relat Res 2009;467(2): 465–72.

28. Vielpeau C, Lebel B, Ardouin L, et al. The dual mobility socket concept: experience with 668 cases. Int Orthop 2011;35(2):225–30.

29. Kershaw CJ, Atkins RM, Dodd CA, et al. Revision total hip arthroplasty for aseptic failure. A review of 276 cases. J Bone Joint Surg Br 1991;73(4): 564–8.

30. Philippot R, Adam P, Reckhaus M, et al. Prevention of dislocation in total hip revision surgery using a dual mobility design. Orthop Traumatol Surg Res 2009;95(6):407–13.

31. Khatod M, Barber T, Paxton E, et al. An analysis of the risk of hip dislocation with a contemporary total joint registry. Clin Orthop Relat Res 2006;447:19–23.

32. Leiber-Wackenheim F, Brunschweiler B, Ehlinger M, et al. Treatment of recurrent THR dislocation using of a cementless dual-mobility cup: a 59 cases series with a mean 8 years' follow-up. Orthop Traumatol Surg Res 2011;97(1):8–13.

33. Guyen O, Pibarot V, Vaz G, et al. Contribution of double-mobility for prosthesis revision for hip instability. J Bone Joint Surg Br 2008;90(Supp II):268.

34. Burgers PT, Van Geene AR, Van den Bekerom MP, et al. Total hip arthroplasty versus hemiarthroplasty for displaced femoral neck fractures in the healthy elderly: a meta-analysis and systematic review of randomized trials. Int Orthop 2012;36(8):1549–60.

35. Iorio R, Healy WL, Lemos DW, et al. Displaced femoral neck fractures in the elderly: outcomes and cost effectiveness. Clin Orthop Relat Res 2001;(383):229–42.

36. Tarasevicius S, Robertsson O, Dobozinskas P, et al. A comparison of outcomes and dislocation rates using dual articulation cups and THA for intracapsular femoral neck fractures. Hip Int 2013;23(1):22–6.

37. Tarasevicius S, Busevicius M, Robertsson O, et al. Dual mobility cup reduces dislocation rate after arthroplasty for femoral neck fracture. BMC Musculoskelet Disord 2010;11:175.

38. Adam P, Philippe R, Ehlinger M, et al. Dual mobility cups hip arthroplasty as a treatment for displaced fracture of the femoral neck in the elderly. A prospective, systematic, multicenter study with specific focus on postoperative dislocation. Orthop Traumatol Surg Res 2012;98(3):296–300.

39. Tarasevicius S, Jermolajevas V, Tarasevicius R, et al. Total hip replacement for the treatment of femoral neck fractures. Long-term results. Medicina 2005; 41(6):465–9.

40. Hamadouche M, Biau DJ, Huten D, et al. The use of a cemented dual mobility socket to treat recurrent dislocation. Clin Orthop Relat Res 2010;468(12): 3248–54.

41. Hailer NP, Weiss RJ, Stark A, et al. Dual-mobility cups for revision due to instability are associated with a low rate of re-revisions due to dislocation: 228 patients from the Swedish Hip Arthroplasty Register. Acta orthopaedica 2012;83(6):566–71.

42. Langlais FL, Ropars M, Gaucher F, et al. Dual mobility cemented cups have low dislocation rates in THA revisions. Clin Orthop Relat Res 2008; 466(2):389–95.

The Local Effects of Metal Corrosion in Total Hip Arthroplasty

H. John Cooper, MD

KEYWORDS

- Adverse local tissue reaction • Corrosion • Metal debris • Modularity • Total hip arthroplasty

KEY POINTS

- Corrosion can occur at any modular junction in total hip arthroplasty (THA), with the potential for release of metal debris and ions into the surrounding local environment.
- The potential for corrosion at a particular modular junction is multifactorial and can depend on factors such as taper geometry, constituent materials, forces applied to the junction, femoral head size, component offset, and method of assembly.
- Local effects of metal corrosion include adverse local tissue reactions (ALTR), component fracture or failure, instability, and osteolysis and loosening.
- Taper corrosion should be considered in the differential diagnosis of hip pain following THA, and appropriate testing should include serum metal levels and cross-sectional imaging such as magnetic resonance imaging to evaluate the surrounding soft tissues.
- Treatment consists of exchange of the modular part responsible for the ALTR when possible, versus revision of the entire component when not possible.

INTRODUCTION

Metal corrosion in total hip arthroplasty (THA) has long been recognized as a theoretical concern that accompanied the introduction of modularity[1] and soon thereafter was documented in numerous retrieval studies of early modular hip components.[2–13] Although there were rare reports of poor clinical outcomes associated with corrosion,[3,11,13,14] any connections between adverse local effects and corrosion were not firmly established at that time.

As design and manufacturing of modular junctions improved through the 1990s and 2000s, most early concerns surrounding corrosion largely disappeared from the literature. However, there has recently been a renewed concern surrounding corrosion in THA, as many groups have reported adverse local tissue reactions (ALTR) and other local complications in association with modular hip components.[15–26] As complications arising from corrosion are being recognized with increasing frequency, it is important for the orthopedic surgeons who perform these procedures and manage these patients postoperatively to understand this process.

This article reviews the important points concluded from retrieval analyses, and explores the multifactorial etiology of corrosion. Local effects of corrosion are reviewed, and diagnostic evaluation and treatment options for patients with metal corrosion discussed.

CORROSION AT MODULAR INTERFACES IN THA

Modularity offers numerous advantages in modern THA. Modular heads and necks offer increased

Disclosure: Dr Cooper is a paid consultant for Smith & Nephew (Memphis, TN).
Department of Orthopaedic Surgery, Lenox Hill Hospital, 130 East 77th Street, 11th Floor, New York, NY 10075, USA
E-mail address: jcooper02@gmail.com

Orthop Clin N Am 45 (2014) 9–18
http://dx.doi.org/10.1016/j.ocl.2013.08.003

intraoperative flexibility to better match native anatomy, leg length, and offset,[27–29] all of which affect stability. Modularity also allows numerous options for head size and choice of bearing surface without requiring a substantial increase in implant inventory. Head-neck modularity further allows the head to be removed at the time of future surgery, either for exposure or to change head size or neck length. In addition, certain implants with modular proximal-stem and mid-stem junctions offer advantages in addressing difficult primary or revision cases. However, as already noted, the addition of these modular junctions does not come without a cost.

Historical Retrieval Analyses

Soon after the introduction of head-neck modularity in THA, numerous retrieval analyses began to report fretting and corrosion at the head-neck junction.[2–13] Early retrievals documented concerns of increased corrosion associated with mixed-metal junctions, resulting from galvanic acceleration between a titanium (Ti) alloy stem and a cobalt-chromium (CoCr) alloy head[2–6]; however, this was challenged in later studies.[7,8,12] Prevalence of corrosion among retrieved specimens ranged from 0% to 57% at 0.5 to 5.5 years,[2–6,8] but was found to be significantly dependent on device and design.[2–8]

Corrosion in Metal-on-Metal THA

Release of metal wear debris from the metal-on-metal (MoM) bearing surface was originally thought to be the major cause in the development of ALTR after large-head MoM THA, as this was the cause for ALTR following hip-resurfacing arthroplasty. However, recent work from multiple investigators has implicated corrosion at the modular head-neck taper interface to be a major contributing factor.[30–41] Given these findings, there is growing concern that the modular taper junction plays a significant role in the failure of large-head MoM THA, although the clinical significance of metal loss from this junction remains somewhat unclear.[30] This additional modular junction may be responsible for the greater elevations in serum metal levels[38] and higher failure rates of large-head MoM THA when compared with hip-resurfacing arthroplasties bearing the same design.[32]

Corrosion in Metal-on-Polyethylene THA

As orthopedic surgeons became more accustomed to seeing adverse reactions to metal debris associated with MoM devices, similar reactions were noted in patients with metal-on-polyethylene bearing surfaces.[15,17–20] Given that the potential for corrosion at this modular head-neck junction had been well established from the retrieval analyses of metal-on-polyethylene THAs discussed previously, these reactions provided clear evidence of a similar mechanism of metal release from modular head-neck junctions (**Fig. 1**), regardless of the bearing surface.

Corrosion at Neck-Body Junctions

Numerous designs of modular neck-body stems, also known as dual-taper stems, have been introduced. Similar to modular head-neck junctions, concerns over corrosion at modular neck-body junctions (**Fig. 2**) were raised soon after these devices were introduced.[42,43] Corrosion at this junction has subsequently been documented in retrieval analyses,[21,22,44] cases of modular neck fracture,[45–47] and reports of ALTR.[16,24] Furthermore, multiple stem designs featuring modular neck junctions from several different manufacturers have been either modified, recalled, or removed from the market after these concerns were noted.

Corrosion at Other Modular Junctions

Concerns over corrosion at stem-sleeve or mid-stem modular junctions were also expressed soon after these devices were introduced.[48] Stem-sleeve devices made from Ti alloy have good mid-term and long-term outcomes reported in both primary and revision settings, although recent reports have raised concerns for fretting and corrosion found at retrieval,[22,49,50] found in association with stem fracture,[50,51] and encountered in junctions with impaired intraoperative disengagement at the time of revision surgery.[52]

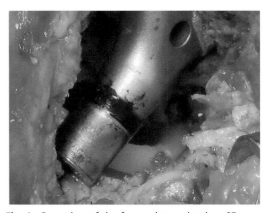

Fig. 1. Corrosion of the femoral trunnion in a 65-year-old woman 3 years following metal-on-polyethylene total hip arthroplasty (THA), seen at the time of revision for adverse local tissue reactions (ALTR).

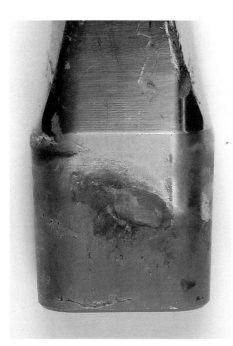

Fig. 2. Severe corrosion at the base of the modular titanium-alloy neck retrieved from a 59-year-old man during femoral revision for severe groin pain secondary to modular neck-body corrosion 4 years following large-head alumina-on-polyethylene THA.

Mid-stem modular junctions can also undergo corrosion, and this process has been found to be more severe at CoCr modular junctions than at Ti modular junctions.[22] A second retrieval study documented severe corrosion in the mating interfaces of mid-stem modular Ti stems with evidence of etching, pitting, delamination, and surface cracking.[53]

In addition, although corrosion is generally thought to be isolated to femoral components, it can also occur in modular acetabular components, and has been correlated with impingement in one recent study.[54]

ETIOLOGY OF CORROSION

Corrosion is fundamentally an electrochemical process of oxidation and reduction reactions. The metals used in THA components are chosen not only because of their high strength, wear resistance, and fatigue resistance, but also because they are highly corrosion-resistant when compared with most other metals because of their ability to form a passive surface film to prevent oxidation.[55] However, owing to the mechanical environment that occurs in vivo, these components are subject to a mechanically assisted corrosion process that can be considerably accelerated when this passive surface film is disrupted through factors such as fretting, micromotion, or other externally applied forces.[55] Furthermore, corrosion is affected by wear through a complex interaction known as tribocorrosion, in which these 2 processes are coupled in a nonlinear manner.[56,57]

Factors Associated with Corrosion

The following factors have been associated with increased mechanical forces, fretting, or corrosion at modular junctions in THA, and are therefore of clinical relevance and concern:

Head size
Several recent studies by multiple independent groups have concluded that head size has a role in the propensity for corrosion at the modular head-neck interface. Frictional torque at the bearing surface, which is transmitted to modular junctions, has been shown to increase with increasing head size from 22 mm to 40 mm in a biomechanical study.[58] Likely because of these increased torsional forces, a recent retrieval study found significantly increased corrosion scores at the head-neck taper interface of 36-mm heads when compared with 28-mm heads.[59] Another recent finite element study has found increased stress and deleterious wear generation at the femoral head-trunnion interface in head sizes larger than 40 mm.[60] Despite this evidence, however, it is clear that corrosion can occur with any size of head, as has been documented in the literature.[15,25]

Neck length and offset
Longer modular heads or necks that offer higher offset increase the load seen at modular junctions,[61] and, as a result, have been shown to lead to higher visual fretting damage in multiple in vitro biomechanical studies and retrieval analyses.[7,62] In addition, a study of large-diameter MoM THAs found that increasing the lever arm through increased offset was the primary factor leading to taper failure.[31]

Head material and bearing surface
Certain head materials are clearly more susceptible than others to fretting and corrosion. CoCr heads have demonstrated greater fretting corrosion when coupled with stainless-steel stems than when coupled with CoCr stems.[62] Furthermore, ceramic heads produce significantly less fretting[63] and corrosion[50] than CoCr alloy heads, and thus have a lower potential for metal release from the modular trunnion. A biomechanical study found significantly greater metal release (11-fold increase in Co and 3-fold increase in Cr) from a

CoCr-CoCr interface when compared with a CoCr-ceramic interface.[63] These protective benefits of ceramics also seem to extend to femoral heads made from oxidized zirconium.[64] However, it must be noted that ceramic heads may not be completely protective against corrosion, as multiple retrieval studies have documented corrosion even in the presence of a ceramic head.[16,50,65]

In addition, the routine use of highly cross-linked polyethylene (XLPE) may also play a role in increasing the risk of fretting and subsequent corrosion at modular taper junctions, as XLPE has been shown in a biomechanical in vitro study to exert a higher frictional torque to the bearing interface than conventional polyethylene.[58]

Stem and trunnion design

Stem design also has an etiologic role in propensity for corrosion. Fully coated cobalt-alloy cementless stems have been shown to have a higher prevalence of intergranular trunnion corrosion in a retrieval analysis of 246 implants,[66] although questions remain as to whether the increased prevalence of corrosion associated with these designs reflects problems in the particular stem as opposed to simple usage patterns at the institutions reporting these cases.

Probably more influential than stem design is trunnion design, which can have considerable effects on the likelihood of corrosion.[39] Flexural rigidity of the trunnion, which depends on taper geometry and the modulus of elasticity of the given metal alloy from which the stem or neck is made, has been found in a large retrieval analysis be among the most important factors responsible for corrosion at the head-neck junction.[8] As a result, stems with a smaller taper geometry and those made from a more flexible alloy may be more prone to fretting and corrosion than stems with larger and stiffer trunnion designs.[67]

Method of assembly

Assembling modular junctions under clean and dry conditions is also important in reducing the risk of corrosion. Modular junctions assembled under contaminated conditions (with bone chips) were found to exhibit greater micromotion than those assembled with a clean interface in an in vitro study.[68] In addition, in a separate biomechanical study dry taper assembly has been found to raise the onset load to fretting corrosion when compared with assembly under wet conditions.[62]

LOCAL EFFECTS OF METAL CORROSION IN THA

Metal release from modular junctions through fretting and corrosion can cause elevated serum metal levels[15,16,69] and particle deposition within local tissues.[10] More concerning, this process can also produce a range of local effects in and around the hip, including the following.

Adverse Local Tissue Reactions

ALTR, which have also been described as pseudotumors, were initially reported as a complication of MoM hip resurfacing and MoM THA,[70,71] with histologic examination of periprosthetic tissues demonstrating large areas of tissue necrosis, chronic inflammatory reaction, and perivascular and diffuse lymphocytic aggregates. Because these reactions arise from a reaction to metal debris, they can also arise from corrosion at modular junctions in THA components.

Svensson and colleagues[14] were the first to report an aggressive soft-tissue reaction following metal-on-polyethylene THA. The patient reported severe pain and weakness 3 years following the index surgery, and on exploration was found to have severe fretting and corrosion at the modular head-neck junction and a large necrotic soft-tissue mass. Following multiple debridements and eventual explantation, the patient was eventually left with a completely denervated leg, a chronically draining wound, and both arterial and venous insufficiency. Three years later, Mathiesen and colleagues[11] described 3 additional cases with similarly extensive soft-tissue reactions and macroscopically visible corrosion at the head-neck interface.

Following these early reports, there were no known additional cases of ALTR secondary to corrosion reported for nearly 2 decades. However, since 2010 there have been several new cases of ALTR described in the setting of corrosion at modular head-neck[15,17–20,25,35,40,41] and neck-body junctions.[16,22,24] Clinical presentations can be variable, but symptoms typically relate to pain secondary to fluid accumulation and tissue destruction, with many patients also describing muscle weakness or a limp.

Instability

Patients with ALTR may not always present with pain. Local tissue destruction with associated abductor weakness can manifest as instability in the setting of mild to no preexisting hip pain, and has been reported in patients with MoM bearings.[72,73] This process can also occur in patients with ALTR secondary to corrosion.[15,25,28,74] If the orthopedic surgeon fails to consider ATLR in the differential diagnosis for recurrent instability, a missed diagnosis might follow.

Loosening and Osteolysis

Local inflammation, mediated by wear debris and ions released from corrosion at the modular junction, can play a role in wear-induced periprosthetic loosening.[75,76] A recent study found that of 114 large-head MoM THAs with corrosion at the modular head-neck junction, 52% demonstrated radiographic evidence of loosening.[41] Other investigators have also reported cases of component loosening in association with corrosion.[11,15]

Corrosion-Induced Implant Fracture

Neck fractures of monolithic stem designs have been associated with corrosion at modular head-neck junctions[3,13,77]; however, these reports are rare and seem to be of minimal clinical concern.

Much more common and more concerning is the potential for modular neck fracture in dual-tapered stems,[45–47,78–82] which is probably the second most common clinical problem arising from metal corrosion after ALTR. This problem has been reported in multiple stem designs, but only in those with a Ti alloy modular neck. The incidence of this complication is clearly design-specific, but has been reported as high as 2.4% with one specific design from Europe.[79] Although most case reports on modular neck fracture have not performed a retrieval analysis, those that have found evidence of corrosion at the site of fracture initiation.[45–47]

In addition to neck fractures, fractures of the femoral stem itself have been reported in association with corrosion at modular stem-sleeve junctions in stem designs with proximal body modularity.[50,51]

Remote and Systemic Effects

Descriptions of systemic manifestations have been sporadically reported in association with elevated metal levels in MoM hip arthroplasty,[83–86] although causality and etiology remain uncertain at present. The literature on systemic effects of taper corrosion is even less clear, with investigators having described findings of depression, weight gain, hemolytic anemia, and local motor and sensory dysfunction[14] as well as decreased appetite and weight loss[20] in patients who also had ALTR secondary to corrosion. As with reports of systemic effects of metallosis following MoM THA, it is difficult to establish causality based on these nonspecific symptoms.

EVALUATION AND MANAGEMENT
Diagnostic Workup

A diagnosis of metal corrosion at modular junctions has not historically been considered in the differential diagnosis of hip pain or dysfunction following THA. As orthopedic surgeons become more familiar with the signs and symptoms of corrosion, and as its apparent prevalence is increasing, it certainly deserves consideration in any diagnostic algorithm.

Patients with metal corrosion may present with symptoms as early as several months after the index arthroplasty procedure[15,16] out to more than a decade.[25] However, mean time to presentation is typically on the order of 1 to 3 years.[15,16,25] Presenting symptoms can be variable, but include groin pain, thigh pain, buttock pain, lateral hip pain, weakness, painless instability, or lower extremity swelling.[15,16,25] ALTR is typically seen more commonly in women than in men,[15,16,25] and several studies of MoM hips have also described a slight gender bias, with females more likely to develop adverse tissue reactions.[87,88]

C-reactive protein (CRP) and erythrocyte sedimentation rate (ESR) are serum inflammatory markers that are recommended in routine evaluation of the painful THA, as they are excellent screening tools for periprosthetic joint infection (PJI). These markers can also be elevated in patients with ALTR from modular taper corrosion. In the larger case series where these values have been examined, ESR and CRP are elevated in approximately half of cases.[15,16,25] Hip aspiration should be obtained in patients with elevated values to further evaluate for the possibility of PJI. Of importance is that the presence of metal and cellular debris and degenerated cells in the synovial fluid aspiration can significantly alter automated cell counts, so a manual cell count should be requested, as this debris may otherwise lead to falsely elevated values.

Serum metal levels (or whole blood levels at institutions where serum levels are not reliably available) should be obtained in every case where a diagnosis of corrosion is being considered. A differential elevation of serum Co over Cr is highly suggestive of a problem at the taper junction, and warrants further investigation.[15,16,25] Reference values for serum Co and Cr that indicate corrosion have not yet been established, but mean values for serum Co of 9.5 ng/mL[15] and 6.0 ng/mL[16] were seen in 2 large case series, with a wide range of values from less than 1 ng/mL to 42.45 ng/mL.[15,16] As these tests have yet to be standardized across different laboratories, and as accurate reference ranges for patients with well-functioning THAs have yet to be established at every laboratory, it is important to interpret values in a clinical context with the patient's presentation.

Specific radiographic findings in patients with metal corrosion are often absent, but some cases can demonstrate subtle findings of periarticular osteolysis and bone resorption (**Fig. 3**).[17,25,26] However, for other complications such as component fracture or loosening, radiographs are the diagnostic test of choice.[45–47,50,51,78–82] Advanced imaging should be obtained in every case where suspicion for ALTR is high or metal levels are elevated. Magnetic resonance imaging (MRI) using one of several metal artifact reduction sequencing (MARS) protocols have high sensitivity in demonstrating fluid collections or soft-tissue masses,[15,16,18,25] and are probably the most important test in the diagnosis of ALTR. Ultrasonography by an experienced technician can be used as a screening test in patients who are unable to tolerate MRI or in regions where MARS MRI is unavailable.[89]

Although certain case reports have described tissue biopsies performed to confirm a diagnosis of ALTR from taper corrosion,[19,20] the specific constellation of clinical symptoms, elevated serum metals, and advanced imaging consistent with fluid collections or soft-tissue masses should be sufficient to establish a diagnosis.

Treatment Options

Management of taper corrosion has received little attention in the literature. Accordingly, there are few definitive recommendations to guide orthopedic surgeons in treating patients with these problems. Because the problem is progressive and worsens with time, revision surgery should be recommended in the setting of clinically significant symptoms, elevated metal levels, and evidence of a local soft-tissue reaction.[15,16,25] The goals of revision surgery for metal corrosion are the same as those of any successful THA revision and include component fixation, stability, and restoration of leg length. In addition, it is imperative for the surgeon to change or remove the modular taper interface where the corrosion is occurring.

Corrosion at the head-neck interface has been managed successfully in the short term with exchange of a modular head to a ceramic femoral head with or without a titanium adapter sleeve,[15,17,19,20,25] thus altering the composition of the taper interface and removing a potential source of Co and Cr debris. Other investigators have reported removal of the entire femoral stem to provide a virgin femoral trunnion.[18] Modular head exchange allows retention of well-fixed femoral components and avoids potential morbidity associated with component removal, which can often require an extended trochanteric osteotomy. Modular head exchange to a ceramic bearing has also been shown to provide a rapid improvement in serum metal levels in the short term,[15] although longer follow-up will be necessary to confirm whether these encouraging early results are durable.

Corrosion at the neck-body interface or other mid-stem modular junctions presents a more challenging problem, as there is no ceramic option available for these interfaces. As a result, it is necessary to remove the stem and revise to a new femoral component without a problematic taper interface.[16,24,26] Because ALTR typically arise from reactions to Co and Cr debris, it is generally recommended that the new revision components avoid CoCr alloy stems or bearing surfaces, and instead use only Ti alloys and ceramic-on-ceramic or ceramic-on-XLPE bearing surfaces, although this recommendation is based on scant evidence to date.

Relatively high rates of major complications (23%–25%) have been reported following revision for metal corrosion.[16,25] Complications that have been reported include periprosthetic fracture,[16,24] recurrent instability,[25] complete sciatic nerve palsy,[25] arterial and venous insufficiency,[14] deep PJI,[25] and chronic wound drainage ultimately leading to resection arthroplasty.[14,18] Many of these complications are related to the extent of tissue damage encountered at revision surgery; accordingly, the high risk of complications could

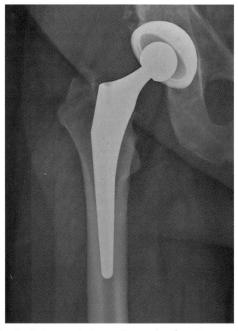

Fig. 3. Anteroposterior radiograph of a 48-year-old man 5 years following metal-on-polyethylene THA, demonstrating bony resorption of the medial neck. At revision for recurrent instability, he was found to have severe corrosion of the femoral trunnion with associated ALTR.

potentially be reduced if diagnosis and management occur before development of aggressive ALTR. In addition, if extensive capsular or muscle damage is seen at the time of revision surgery, there should be a low threshold for using a constrained liner,[15,16,25] particularly if there is compromise of the abductor mechanism.

SUMMARY

Metal corrosion can occur at any modular junction in THA, although it most commonly occurs at the modular head-neck or neck-body junction. Corrosion can occur regardless of the type of bearing surface, but represents a major failure mechanism of large-head MoM THA. When present, corrosion can cause a spectrum of local effects, the most common of which are ALTR and component fracture. ALTR may manifest as pain, weakness, swelling, or recurrent instability without an otherwise obvious cause. The precise etiology of these biological reactions remains unclear, but relates to release of metal debris from corrosion at the modular junction and depends on several mechanical factors intrinsic to the taper junction. Diagnosis of metal corrosion can be made from a constellation of findings, including elevated serum metal levels and the presence of local tissue reaction on MARS MRI. Treatment is directed at removing or changing the interface of the problematic modular junction to stop the ongoing metal release, and revision surgery has a relatively high rate of major complications.

Increased awareness of the potential for metal corrosion at modular junctions will allow orthopedic surgeons the potential for earlier diagnosis and treatment of ALTR, which could thereby prevent ongoing tissue destruction around problematic implants. In addition, implant choices can be made that reduce the risk of taper corrosion by using modular heads that decrease the risk of trunnion corrosion, and by reserving modular implants for complex primary and revision cases that demand their use.

Mechanically assisted corrosion of THA implants will continue to be a concern for the foreseeable future. As a result, prosthetic designs and materials to mitigate or eliminate the source of metal release should be a strong consideration as the orthopedic device industry moves forward.

REFERENCES

1. Lucas L, Buchanan R, Lemons J. Investigations on the galvanic corrosion of multialloy total hip prostheses. J Biomed Mater Res 1981;15:731–47.

2. Collier JP, Surprenant VA, Jensen RE, et al. Corrosion between the components of modular femoral hip prostheses. J Bone Joint Surg Br 1992;74:511.

3. Collier J, Mayor M, Williams I, et al. The tradeoffs associated with modular hip prostheses. Clin Orthop Relat Res 1995;91–101.

4. Collier J, Surprenant V, Jensen R, et al. Corrosion at the interface of cobalt-alloy heads on titanium-alloy stems. Clin Orthop Relat Res 1991;305–12.

5. Cook S, Barrack R, Baffes G, et al. Wear and corrosion of modular interfaces in total hip replacements. Clin Orthop Relat Res 1994;80–8.

6. Cook S, Barrack R, Clemow A. Corrosion and wear at the modular interface of uncemented femoral stems. J Bone Joint Surg Br 1994;76:68–72.

7. Brown SA, Flemming CA, Kawalec JS, et al. Fretting corrosion accelerates crevice corrosion of modular hip tapers. J Appl Biomater 1995;6:19–26.

8. Goldberg J, Gilbert J, Jacobs J, et al. A multicenter retrieval study of the taper interfaces of modular hip prostheses. Clin Orthop Relat Res 2002;149–61.

9. Lieberman J, Rimnac C, Garvin K, et al. An analysis of the head-neck taper interface in retrieved hip prostheses. Clin Orthop Relat Res 1994;162–7.

10. Urban R, Jacobs J, Gilbert J, et al. Migration of corrosion products from modular hip prostheses. Particle microanalysis and histopathological findings. J Bone Joint Surg Am 1994;76:1345–59.

11. Mathiesen EB, Lindgren JU, Blomgren GG, et al. Corrosion of modular hip prostheses. J Bone Joint Surg Br 1991;73:569–75.

12. Gilbert JL, Buckley CA, Jacobs JJ. In vivo corrosion of modular hip prosthesis components in mixed and similar metal combinations. The effect of crevice, stress, motion, and alloy coupling. J Biomed Mater Res 1993;27:1533–44.

13. Gilbert J, Buckley C, Jacobs J, et al. Intergranular corrosion-fatigue failure of cobalt-alloy femoral stems. A failure analysis of two implants. J Bone Joint Surg Am 1994;76:110–5.

14. Svensson O, Mathiesen E, Reinholt F, et al. Formation of a fulminant soft-tissue pseudotumor after uncemented hip arthroplasty. A case report. J Bone Joint Surg Am 1988;70:1238–42.

15. Cooper HJ, Della Valle CJ, Berger R, et al. Corrosion at the head-neck taper as a cause for adverse local tissue reactions in total hip arthroplasty. J Bone Joint Surg Am 2012;94(18):1655–61.

16. Cooper HJ, Urban RM, Wixson RL, et al. Adverse local tissue reaction arising from corrosion at the femoral neck-body junction in a dual-taper stem with a cobalt-chromium modular neck. J Bone Joint Surg Am 2013;95:865–72.

17. Meftah M, Nicolaou N, Rodriguez JA. Metal allergy response to femoral head-neck corrosion after total hip replacement. Current Orthopaedic Practice 2010;21:530.

18. Lindgren J, Brismar B, Wikstrom A. Adverse reaction to metal release from a modular metal-on-polyethylene hip prosthesis. J Bone Joint Surg Br 2011;93:1427–30.

19. Mao X, Tay G, Godbolt D, et al. Pseudotumor in a well-fixed metal-on-polyethylene uncemented hip arthroplasty. J Arthroplasty 2012;27:493.e13–7.

20. Walsh A, Nikolaou V, Antoniou J. Inflammatory pseudotumor complicating metal-on-highly cross-linked polyethylene total hip arthroplasty. J Arthroplasty 2012;27:324.e5–8.

21. Kop AM, Swarts E. Corrosion of a hip stem with a modular neck taper junction: a retrieval study of 16 cases. J Arthroplasty 2009;24:1019–23.

22. Kop AM, Keogh C, Swarts E. Proximal component modularity in THA—at what cost?: an implant retrieval study. Clin Orthop Relat Res 2012;470: 1885–94.

23. Kretzer JP, Jakubowitz E, Krachler M, et al. Metal release and corrosion effects of modular neck total hip arthroplasty. Int Orthop 2009;33:1531–6.

24. Gill IPS, Webb J, Sloan K, et al. Corrosion at the neck-stem junction as a cause of metal ion release and pseudotumour formation. J Bone Joint Surg Br 2012;94:895–900.

25. Cooper HJ, Della Valle CJ, Jacobs JJ. Biologic implications of taper corrosion in total hip arthroplasty. Semin Arthroplasty 2012;23(4):273–8.

26. Meneghini RM, Hallab NJ, Jacobs JJ. Evaluation and treatment of painful total hip arthroplasties with modular metal taper junctions. Orthopedics 2012;35:386–91.

27. Archibeck MJ, Cummins T, Carothers J, et al. A comparison of two implant systems in restoration of hip geometry in arthroplasty. Clin Orthop Relat Res 2011;469:443–6.

28. Sariali E, Mouttret A, Pasquier G, et al. Accuracy of reconstruction of the hip using computerized three-dimensional pre-operative planning and a cementless modular neck. J Bone Joint Surg Br 2009;91: 333–40.

29. Duwelius PJ, Hartzband MA, Burkhart R, et al. Clinical results of a modular neck hip system: hitting the "bull's-eye" more accurately. Am J Orthop 2010;39(Suppl 10):2–6.

30. Matthies AK, Racasan R, Bills P, et al. Material loss at the taper junction of retrieved large head metal-on-metal total hip replacements. J Orthop Res 2013 [Epub ahead of print; PMID: 23918742].

31. Langton DJ, Sidaginamale R, Lord JK, et al. Taper junction failure in large-diameter metal-on-metal bearings. Bone Joint Res 2012;1:56–63.

32. Langton D, Jameson S, Joyce T, et al. Accelerating failure rate of the ASR total hip replacement. J Bone Joint Surg Br 2011;93:1011–6.

33. Langton D, Jameson S, Joyce T, et al. Early failure of metal-on-metal bearings in hip resurfacing and large-diameter total hip replacement: a consequence of excess wear. J Bone Joint Surg Br 2010;92:38.

34. Kwon YM, Jacobs JJ, MacDonald SJ, et al. Evidence-based understanding of management perils for metal-on-metal hip arthroplasty patients. J Arthroplasty 2012;27(Suppl 8):20–5.

35. Natu S, Sidaginamale RP, Gandhi J, et al. Adverse reactions to metal debris: histopathological features of periprosthetic soft tissue reactions seen in association with failed metal on metal hip arthroplasties. J Clin Pathol 2012;65:409–18.

36. Bolland B, Culliford D, Langton D, et al. High failure rates with a large-diameter hybrid metal-on-metal total hip replacement: clinical, radiological and retrieval analysis. J Bone Joint Surg Br 2011;93:608.

37. Chana R, Esposito C, Campbell P, et al. Mixing and matching causing taper wear: corrosion associated with pseudotumour formation. J Bone Joint Surg Br 2012;94:281–6.

38. Garbuz D, Tanzer M, Greidanus N, et al. The John Charnley Award: metal-on-metal hip resurfacing versus large-diameter head metal-on-metal total hip arthroplasty: a randomized clinical trial. Clin Orthop Relat Res 2010;468:318–25.

39. Nassif NA, Nawabi DH, Stoner K, et al. Taper design affects failure of large-head metal-on-metal total hip replacements. Clin Orthop Relat Res 2013 [Epub ahead of print; PMID 23801060].

40. Fricka KB, Ho H, Peace WJ, et al. Metal-on-metal local tissue reaction is associated with corrosion of the head taper junction. J Arthroplasty 2012; 27(Suppl 8):26–31.e1.

41. Meyer H, Mueller T, Goldau G, et al. Corrosion at the cone/taper interface leads to failure of large-diameter metal-on-metal total hip arthroplasties. Clin Orthop Relat Res 2012;470:3101–8.

42. Viceconti M, Ruggeri O, Toni A, et al. Design-related fretting wear modular neck hip prosthesis. J Biomed Mater Res 1996;30:181–6.

43. Viceconti M, Baleani M, Squarzoni S, et al. Fretting wear in a modular neck hip prosthesis. J Biomed Mater Res 1997;35:207–16.

44. Levine BR, Hall DJ, Urban RM, et al. Fretting corrosion and fracture of the modular neck-body junctions in hip replacement femoral components. AAOS Annual Meeting, New Orleans, LA, March, 2010.

45. Atwood SA, Patten EW, Bozic KJ, et al. Corrosion-induced fracture of a double-modular hip prosthesis: a case report. J Bone Joint Surg Am 2010; 92:1522–5.

46. Dangles CJ, Alstetter CJ. Failure of the modular neck in a total hip arthroplasty. J Arthroplasty 2010;25:1169.e5–7.

47. Wright G, Sporer S, Urban R, et al. Fracture of a modular femoral neck after total hip arthroplasty:

a case report. J Bone Joint Surg Am 2010;92: 1518–21.

48. Bobyn JD, Tanzer M, Krygier JJ, et al. Concerns with modularity in total hip arthroplasty. Clin Orthop Relat Res 1994;298:27–38.

49. Mehran N, North T, Laker M. Failure of a modular hip implant at the stem-sleeve interface. Orthopedics 2013;36:e978–81.

50. Huot Carlson JC, Van Citters DW, Currier JH, et al. Femoral stem fracture and in vivo corrosion of retrieved modular femoral hips. J Arthroplasty 2012;27:1389–96.e1.

51. Patel A, Bliss J, Calfee RP, et al. Modular femoral stem-sleeve junction failure after primary total hip arthroplasty. J Arthroplasty 2009;24:1143.e1–5.

52. Fraitzl CR, Moya LE, Castellani L, et al. Corrosion at the stem-sleeve interface of a modular titanium alloy femoral component as a reason for impaired disengagement. J Arthroplasty 2011;26:113–9, 119.e1.

53. Rodrigues DC, Urban RM, Jacobs JJ, et al. In vivo severe corrosion and hydrogen embrittlement of retrieved modular body titanium alloy hip-implants. J Biomed Mater Res B Appl Biomater 2009;88: 206–19.

54. Kligman M, Furman BD, Padgett DE, et al. Impingement contributes to backside wear and screw-metallic shell fretting in modular acetabular cups. J Arthroplasty 2007;22:258–64.

55. Jacobs JJ, Gilbert JL, Urban RM. Corrosion of metal orthopaedic implants. J Bone Joint Surg Am 1998;80:268–82.

56. Mathew MT, Runa MJ, Laurent M, et al. Tribocorrosion behavior of CoCrMo alloy for hip prosthesis as a function of loads: a comparison between two testing systems. Wear 2011;271:1210–9.

57. Mathew MT, Srinivasa Pai P, Pourzal R, et al. Significance of tribocorrosion in biomedical applications: overview and current status. Adv Tribology 2009 [Article ID: 250986].

58. Burroughs BR, Muratoglu OK, Bragdon CR, et al. In vitro comparison of frictional torque and torsional resistance of aged conventional gamma-in-nitrogen sterilized polyethylene versus aged highly cross-linked polyethylene articulating against head sizes larger than 32 mm. Acta Orthop 2006;77:710–8.

59. Dyrkacz RM, Brandt JM, Ojo OA, et al. The influence of head size on corrosion and fretting behaviour at the head-neck interface of artificial hip joints. J Arthroplasty 2013;28:1036–40.

60. Elkins J, Callaghan J, Brown TD. Possible failure due to wear at the trunnion interface in large diameter metal-on-metal total hips: a finite element analysis. ORS, Annual Meeting. San Antonio, TX, January, 2013.

61. Doehring TC, Rubash HE, Dore DE. Micromotion measurements with hip center and modular neck length alterations. Clin Orthop Relat Res 1999; 362:230–9.

62. Gilbert J, Mehta M, Pinder B. Fretting crevice corrosion of stainless steel stem-CoCr femoral head connections: comparisons of materials, initial moisture, and offset length. J Biomed Mater Res B Appl Biomater 2009;88:162–73.

63. Hallab NJ, Messina C, Skipor A, et al. Differences in the fretting corrosion of metal-metal and ceramic-metal modular junctions of total hip replacements. J Orthop Res 2004;22:250–9.

64. Tsai S, Heuer D, Pawar V, et al. Fretting corrosion testing of various femoral head/taper material combinations. Society for Biomaterials, 30th Annual Meeting. Memphis, TN, April, 2005.

65. Kurtz SM, Kocagöz SB, Hanzlik JA, et al. Do ceramic femoral heads reduce taper fretting corrosion in hip arthroplasty? A retrieval study. Clin Orthop Relat Res 2013 [Epub ahead of print; PMID: 23761174].

66. Urban R, Hall D, Gilbert J, et al. Have fretting and corrosion been reduced in contemporary head/neck modular junctions? American Academy of Orthopaedic Surgeons, Annual Meeting. San Francisco, CA, March, 2012.

67. Porter D, Urban R, Jacobs JJ, et al. Flexural rigidity of various trunnion designs in modular hip stems: a biomechanical and historical analysis. International Society for Technology in Arthroplasty, 26th Annual Meeting. Palm Beach, FL, October, 2013.

68. Jauch S, Huber G, Hoenig E, et al. Influence of material coupling and assembly condition on the magnitude of micromotion at the stem-neck interface of a modular hip endoprosthesis. J Biomech 2011;44:1747–51.

69. Jacobs J, Urban R, Gilbert J, et al. Local and distant products from modularity. Clin Orthop Relat Res 1995;94–105.

70. Pandit H, Glyn-Jones S, Mclardy-Smith P, et al. Pseudotumours associated with metal-on-metal hip resurfacings. J Bone Joint Surg Br 2008;90:847–51.

71. Willert HG, Buchhorn GH, Fayyazi A, et al. Metal-on-metal bearings and hypersensitivity in patients with artificial hip joints. A clinical and histomorphological study. J Bone Joint Surg Am 2005;87:28–36.

72. Theruvil B, Vasukutty N, Hancock N, et al. Dislocation of large diameter metal-on-metal bearings an indicator of metal reaction? J Arthroplasty 2011; 26:832–7.

73. Killampalli VV, Reading AD. Late instability of bilateral metal on metal hip resurfacings due to progressive local tissue effects. Hip Int 2009;19:287–91.

74. Leopold SS, Silverton CD, Urban RM, et al. Late dislocations associated with corrosion at the head-neck interface of modular THA components. American Academy of Orthopaedic Surgeons, 2001 Annual Meeting. San Francisco, CA.

75. Korovessis P, Petsinis G, Repanti M, et al. Metallosis after contemporary metal-on-metal total hip arthroplasty. Five to nine-year follow-up. J Bone Joint Surg Am 2006;88(6):1183–91.

76. Jacobs JJ, Hallab NJ. Loosening and osteolysis associated with metal-on-metal bearings: a local effect of metal hypersensitivity? J Bone Joint Surg Am 2006;88(6):1171–2.

77. Botti TP, Gent J, Martell JM, et al. Trunnion fracture of a fully porous-coated femoral stem. J Arthroplasty 2005;20:943–5.

78. Ellman MB, Levine BR. Fracture of the modular femoral neck component in total hip arthroplasty. J Arthroplasty 2013;28:196.e1–5.

79. Grupp TM, Weik T, Bloemer W, et al. Modular titanium alloy neck adapter failures in hip replacement—failure mode analysis and influence of implant material. BMC Musculoskelet Disord 2010;11:3.

80. Skendzel JG, Blaha JD, Urquhart AG. Total hip arthroplasty modular neck failure. J Arthroplasty 2011;26:338.e1–4.

81. Sotereanos NG, Sauber TJ, Tupis TT. Modular femoral neck fracture after primary total hip arthroplasty. J Arthroplasty 2013;28:196.e7–9.

82. Wilson DAJ, Dunbar MJ, Amirault JD, et al. Early failure of a modular femoral neck total hip arthroplasty component. J Bone Joint Surg Am 2010; 92:1514–7.

83. Ikeda T, Takahashi K, Kabata T, et al. Polyneuropathy caused by cobalt-chromium metallosis after total hip replacement. Muscle Nerve 2010;42: 140–3.

84. Oldenburg M, Wegner R, Baur X. Severe cobalt intoxication due to prosthesis wear in repeated total hip arthroplasty. J Arthroplasty 2009;24:825. e15–20.

85. Rizzetti MC, Liberini P, Zarattini G, et al. Loss of sight and sound. Could it be the hip? Lancet 2009;373:1052.

86. Tower SS. Arthroprosthetic cobaltism: neurological and cardiac manifestations in two patients with metal-on-metal arthroplasty: a case report. J Bone Joint Surg Am 2010;92:2847–51.

87. Latteier MJ, Berend KR, Lombardi AV Jr, et al. Gender is a significant factor for failure of metal-on-metal total hip arthroplasty. J Arthroplasty 2011;26(Suppl 6):19–23.

88. Glyn-Jones S, Pandit H, Kwon YM, et al. Risk factors for inflammatory pseudotumour formation following hip resurfacing. J Bone Joint Surg Br 2009;91(12):1566–74.

89. Garbuz DS, Hargreaves BA, Duncan CP, et al. The John Charnley Award: diagnostic accuracy of MRI versus ultrasound for detecting pseudotumors in asymptomatic metal-on-metal THA. Clin Orthop Relat Res 2013 [Epub ahead of print; PMID 23868425].

The Rationale for Short Uncemented Stems in Total Hip Arthroplasty

Ronak M. Patel, MD, S. David Stulberg, MD*

KEYWORDS

- Short stem implants • Metaphyseal-engaging implants • Uncemented total hip arthroplasty

KEY POINTS

- Metaphyseal fit and ingrowth can provide both rotational and axial stability without distal diaphyseal support.
- Bone remodeling on radiographic analysis of short stems of various designs show endosteal condensation and cortical hypertrophy in the proximal metaphyseal region of the femur.
- Functional Harris Hip Scores (HHS) and Western Ontario and McMaster Universities Arthritis Index (WOMAC) pain scores are equivalent in patients with metaphyseal-engaging short stems compared with stems of conventional length.
- Short stem metaphyseal-engaging implants enhance the preservation of proximal femoral bone stock as well as provide an adaptive alternative in minimally invasive anterior approaches.
- Metaphyseal-engaging short stems provide an alternative to bone preservation procedures with reproducible and reliable radiographic and clinical outcomes while maintaining a short learning curve.

INTRODUCTION

Total hip arthroplasty (THA) has proved clinically and functionally successful in the treatment of end-stage degenerative joint disease of the hip.[1–8] Porous-coated, uncemented femoral stems were introduced for use in THA in the early 1980s. Uncemented implants rely on diaphyseal or metaphyseal contact and, ultimately, bone fixation to ingrowth or ongrowth surfaces to provide long-term stability and dependable clinical results.[3,9–19] Uncemented, porous femoral implants are now routinely used in virtually all patients undergoing primary THA. Uncemented femoral components with a variety of shapes, metallurgy, and surface treatment have been developed to address the broad spectrum of proximal femoral morphology.[12,17,20–24]

Despite the documented success of these implants, current uncemented stems are used in patients whose size, age, level of physical activity, and bone quality present particular challenges for uncemented fixation technologies. These

Conflict of Interest: One or more of the authors (S.D. Stulberg) has received royalties from Aesculap and stock or stock options from Stryker and Johnson & Johnson and serves as a paid consultant to Aesculap, Innomed, Stryker, and Zimmer. The remaining authors certify that they have no commercial associations (consultancies, stock ownership, equity interest, patent/licensing arrangements, etc.) that might pose a conflict of interest in connection with this article.

No benefits in any form have been received or will be received from a commercial party related directly or indirectly to the subject of this article.

Department of Orthopaedic Surgery, Feinberg School of Medicine, Northwestern University, 676 N. St. Clair, Suite #1350, Chicago, IL 60611, USA

* Corresponding author. Northwestern Orthopaedic Institute, LLC, 680 North Lakeshore Drive, Suite 924.

E-mail address: jointsurg@northwestern.edu

Orthop Clin N Am 45 (2014) 19–31

http://dx.doi.org/10.1016/j.ocl.2013.08.007

challenges include (1) the preservation of proximal femoral bone stock; (2) the potential need for effective, femoral component revision; (3) proximal-distal mismatch; and (4) the ability to insert implants safely, securely, and reproducibly with specific surgical approaches (eg, the direct anterior) that are currently being evaluated and promoted.

Short stem uncemented femoral implants have been developed to address some of these challenges while maintaining the current level of success achieved by uncemented implants of conventional length (**Fig. 1**). Short stem implants have been defined as 120 mm in length or less, which approximately correlates to the metadiaphyseal junction of the proximal femur.[25]

The purposes of this article are to (1) explain the evolution to short stem design, (2) describe the rationale and types of short stem implants, (3) provide the benefits of short stem implants, and (4) summarize the clinical results with these implants.

EVOLUTION TO SHORT STEM DESIGN

To understand the evolution of uncemented THA to short stem implants, femoral implant design and stability must first be reviewed. Successful THA relies on initial and long-term rotational and axial stability. The diaphyseal portion (cylindrical or tapered) of the femoral implant contributes to the initial stability. Cylindrical, extensively porous-coated implants (eg, AML) achieve durable fixation

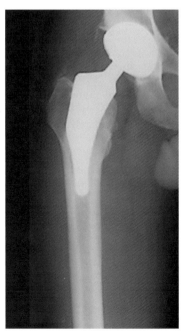

Fig. 1. Young active man with Dorr type A bone.

but can be associated with stress shielding and thigh pain. Cylindrical implants without porous-coated stems achieve varying degrees of initial axial and rotational stability through contact points in the diaphysis but rely on metaphyseal bone contact to enhance their initial rotational stability. Furthermore, these implants seek long-term fixation and stability through bone ingrowth or on-growth at the metaphysis. Long-term clinical results of these implants have been satisfactory and reliable with an overall lower incidence of thigh pain and proximal stress shielding relative to their extensively coated counterparts. Early concerns with a cylindrical diaphysis, however, inspired investigators to produce tapered stems.

Tapered uncemented implants achieve primary axial fixation through a 3-point contact mechanism with the creation, and ultimate relaxation, of hoop stresses between a tapered stem and cylindrical femur. Rotational stability is achieved in the proximal femur through surface treatment, various shape geometries, and overall fit and fill. Secondary fixation depends on the extent of contact between the ingrowth/ongrowth surfaces of the implant and metaphyseal bone. Many studies have established the long-term clinical and radiographic reliability and durability of tapered femoral implants. These stems have been associated with little thigh pain compared with cylindrical stems.

In these designs, the tapered or uncoated cylindrical diaphyseal portion provides primary axial stability but varying degrees of rotational stability. Rather, rotational stability is attained from metaphyseal bone-implant contact.

DESIGN RATIONALE AND TYPES OF UNCEMENTED SHORT STEM METAPHYSEAL-ENGAGING FEMORAL IMPLANTS

Short stem metaphyseal-engaging implants achieve secure initial fixation in the metaphysis, theoretically making the axial and rotational stability provided by the diaphyseal portion of the femoral implant negligible. Metaphyseal ingrowth or on-growth secures long-term fixation, with the pattern of bone implant contact varying by implant design. A variety of implants have been introduced over the past few years, leading to the development of a classification system by McTighe and colleagues.[25] The 3 main types of short stem implants are

1. Metaphyseal stabilized (standard neck resection) (**Fig. 2**A)
2. Neck stabilized (femoral neck sparing) (see **Fig. 2**B)
3. Head stabilized (resurfacing-type procedures) (see **Fig. 2**C)

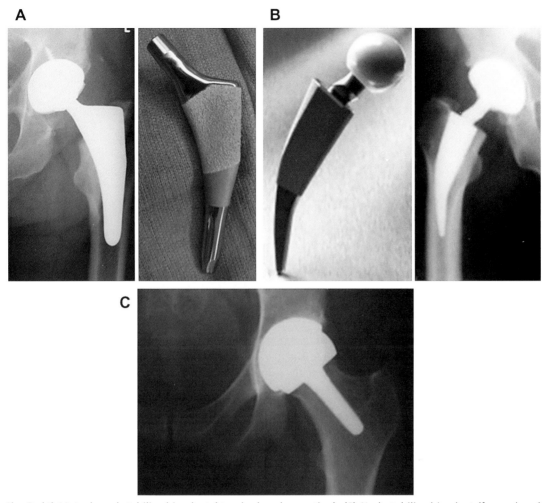

Fig. 2. (*A*) Metaphyseal-stabilized implant (standard neck resection). (*B*) Neck-stabilized implant (femoral neck sparing). (*C*) Head-stabilized implant.

Standard neck resection short stem implants can further be classified into (a) anatomic and (b) wedge fit implants. These implants also tend to be shortened versions of conventional uncemented implants. Femoral neck-sparing or neck-preserving implants instead have unique design features to accommodate the native anteversion of the femoral neck. Head-stabilized short stem implants commission a completely different surgical technique and necessitate specific clinical indications; thus, they are not discussed in this article.

Femoral neck-sparing or high femoral neck resection designs seek to optimize proximal load transfer by engaging solely the femoral neck and the metaphysis. A more proximal and horizontal femoral neck osteotomy produces an oval-shaped intramedullary opening compared with a standard cut, which offers a broad opening

(**Fig. 3**). Studies have shown greater resistance to torsional stresses with these high-neck osteotomies.[26–28] The concept of femoral neck preservation in uncemented designs has been well described since the earliest days of arthroplasty.[29,30] Proponents of this concept have suggested improved bone and soft tissue preservation. Moreover, soft tissue preservation enhances implant fixation, reduces surgical morbidity, improves abductor function, and preserves bone stock for potential future surgery.

Santori and Santori[31] reported satisfactory midterm results in a high femoral neck resection short stem implant. They performed a complete clinical review at a mean interval of 8 years in their cohort of patients under the age of 60 who underwent THA. Despite other encouraging results reported by the developers of uncemented femoral components inserted with high femoral neck

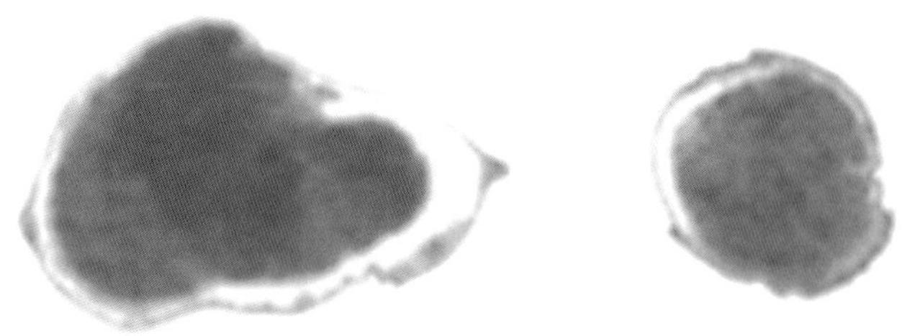

Fig. 3. Cross-sections of osteotomy levels for standard neck versus femoral neck-sparing implants designs.

resection, widespread use of these devices has not yet occurred.

Several reasons have been proposed for the slow adoption of this concept:

1. The surgical technique for inserting stems of this design is different from and potentially more difficult than more standard neck resection approaches. The long retained femoral neck can make exposure of the acetabulum difficult.
2. Accurate, reproducible alignment of the femoral stem within the diaphysis may be difficult to accomplish given the native anteversion of neck shaft.
3. The small surface area of bone at the proximal femoral neck makes restoration of accurate leg length and avoidance of lengthening of the extremity difficult to achieve.
4. The high-neck resection limits exposure of the metaphysis and may reduce the extent and reliability with which metaphyseal fit and contact can be achieved.
5. The combination of high-neck resection and short stems may be associated with an increased incidence of proximal femoral fractures.
6. A high femoral neck resection may result in increased bone-bone impingement and, subsequently, a reduction in range of motion.

Initial experimentation with femoral neck preservation short stem implants may have been considered a radical shift in paradigm at the time. Recent renewed interest in these stems is largely due to a natural progression of uncemented femoral components from cylindrical to tapered to shortened designs. Design teams continue to develop high-neck resection implants based on encouraging results from original designs and aim to address some of the design flaws (discussed previously) (**Fig. 4**). For example, the Fitmore stem (Zimmer, Warsaw, Indiana) has variability in its curve to allow for greater medial calcar contact for enhanced stability (**Fig. 5**). Development of these

devices is spurred by a renewed interest in the use of the direct anterior approach for THA, the desire for surgical and implant approaches that minimize soft tissue and bone trauma, and a concern about proximal bone preservation and positive bone remodeling.

Standard neck resection metaphyseal-engaging short stem implants tend to be shortened versions of commercially available conventional-length uncemented femoral implants (**Fig. 6**). These stems have shortened tapered or cylindrical diaphyseal-reaching stems and a wide variety of metaphyseal shapes. The 2 main categories of metaphyseal shapes include 2-D or 3-D taper shapes that achieve 2-point wedge fixation in the metaphysis and anatomic shapes that seek to fit and fill the metaphysis. Theoretic studies have shown that the use of a lateral flare configuration reduces distal femoral stress transfer in conventional-length uncemented femoral components by engaging the proximal lateral, medial, and anterior cortices.[32,33] Use of this rationale has extended into short stem designs.

Proponents of these short stem designs state the proximal metaphyesal fixation achieved is adequate for initial and long-term stability. Various designs have been shown to have reliable fixation and successful clinical and radiographic outcomes up to 8 years postoperatively.[29,34–36] Two-point wedge designs attempt to achieve contact and fit at the metaphyseal-diaphyseal junction. Although these implants can be tapered in 2 or 3 dimensions, the wedge-fit is primarily 2-point at the medial and lateral cortices (**Fig. 7**). Anterior and/or posterior endosteal contact is variable on design. Similarly, anatomic implants attempt fit and fill the metaphysis—in the coronal or sagittal planes or in both.

Recently, a finite element analysis was completed in a composite bone model evaluating uncemented femoral stem length on primary stability.[37] No significant reduction in stability was observed from reducing stem length from 146 mm to 105 mm; furthermore, decreasing

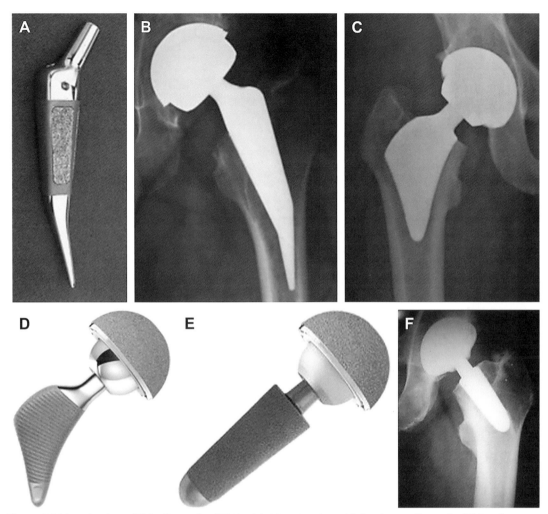

Fig. 4. (*A*) Mayo implant. (*B*) Radiograph of THA with Mayo Implant. (*C*) Proxima radiograph. (*D*) Proxima stem. (*E*) Silent implant and (*F*) radiograph.

stem length further did not lead to micromotion that would inhibit osteointegration.[38] Furthermore, 2-year migration analysis of a metaphyseal anchored short stem implant using Ein Bild Roentgen Analyse femoral component analysis showed subsidence rates and patterns of stability comparable to conventional-length uncemented implants.[39] Although long-term studies remain the gold standard in joint arthroplasty, migration analysis allows prediction of implant survival.

Preservation of proximal femoral bone stock is becoming increasingly important because THA is performed in younger, more active patients. Distal bone-implant fixation can lead to proximal femoral stress shielding and subsequent bone loss. Arno and colleagues[40] completed a cadaveric evaluation of femoral strain with the use of uncemented femoral components with 3 different stem lengths. As the stem length increased, there

was a typical pattern of increased distal strain and decreased proximal femoral strain. This pattern can, theoretically, by Wolff's law, contribute to stress shielding in the proximal femur. These investigators concluded that although the stemless component best matched the strain pattern in a native femur, the ultrashort implant (one-third length of standard Revelation Lateral Flare, DJO Surgical, Austin, Texas) performed close to the stemless design. A proposed benefit of short stem femoral implants is optimal proximal bone remodeling. Although roentgen stereophotogrammetric and dual energy x-ray absorptiometry (DEXA) analysis are considered gold standards in accurate measurement of bone mass surrounding a prosthesis, many investigators report appreciable changes on radiographic analysis. In comparison with conventional-length uncemented femoral implants, short stem implants have less

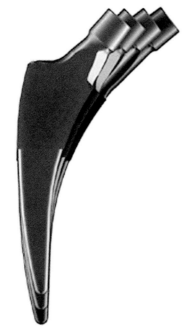

Fig. 5. Zimmer Fitmore short stem implant.

bone resorption.[41] Chen and colleagues[41] found an average bone loss of 3.3% in DEXA analysis of the Mayo Conservative stem (Zimmer, Warsaw, Indiana). The average bone resorption found in the literature is 20%, with an autopsy retrieval study showing 42.1% loss proximally and a gradual decline distally.[42,43]

THEORETIC ADVANTAGES OF SHORT STEM FEMORAL IMPLANTS
Ease and Safety of Revision Surgery

The proximal bone resorption from stress shielding not only results in increased susceptibility to particle-induced osteolysis but also can complicate revision surgery.[41] The senior author has had a particular interest in short stem metaphyseal-engaging femoral implants. Recent use of a short stem modular femoral neck prosthesis (ABG II, Stryker, Mahwah, New Jersey) led to adverse local soft tissue reaction in a small percentage of patients from corrosion at the trunion of the femoral head-neck junction.[44] Similar soft tissue responses have been seen in modular femoral neck prostheses of conventional length (Rejuvenate, Stryker, Mahwah, New Jersey). Ultimately, revision surgery with component extraction and exchange to nonmodular prosthesis is recommended. The 2 case examples of these complications highlight potential benefits of revision surgery with a short stem femoral implant compared with a conventional-length implant.

Revision of a short stem implant

The posterolateral incision and exposure from the primary THA surgery was used and extended both

A   **B**   **C**

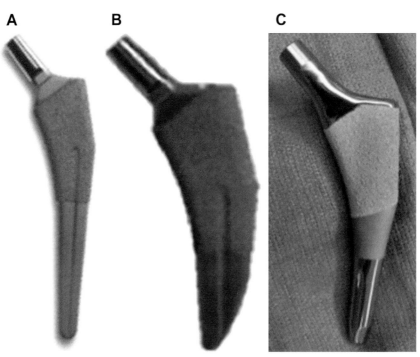

Fig. 6. (*A*) Taperloc. (*B*) Microplasty. (*C*) Citation short.

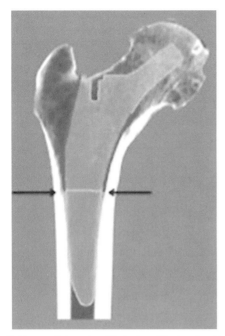

Fig. 7. Two-point wedge fit design. The implant is designed to contact the medial and lateral cortices at the metaphyseal-diaphyseal junction.

proximally and distally. The hip was dislocated and granulomatous tissue was excised. The head and modular tapered neck were removed without difficulty. The cobalt-chromium stem of the ABG implant appeared well aligned and well fixed. A pencil-tip burr created an opening along the shoulder of the femoral component, which allowed for a series of flexible osteotomes to be inserted. After circumferential wedging with the osteotomes, the implant extractor tool was used to remove the femoral component while preserving as much bone as possible. The quality of bone of the proximal femur was good. There was little bone loss. The decision was made to insert a nonmodular ABG implant. The femur was broached sequentially to 1 size up from the original modular ABG implant. After trial reduction and range of motion, the real implant was placed with solid circumferential fixation (**Fig. 8**).

Revision of a conventional-length implant
The posterolateral incision and exposure from the primary THA surgery was used and extended both proximally and distally. The hip was dislocated and granulomatous tissue was excised. The head and modular tapered neck were removed without difficulty. The titanium stem of the Rejuvenate implant was visualized and appeared well fixed. Initially, a 2.3-mm burr was used to open the proximal interface. A thin saw blade was then inserted into the

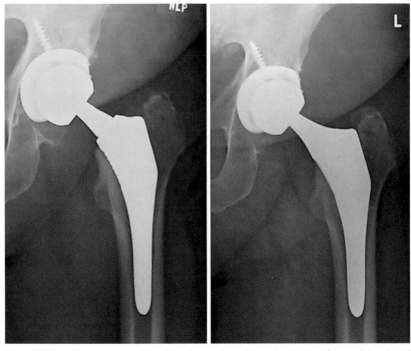

Fig. 8. Prerevision (*left*) and postrevision (*right*) radiographs with a short stem femoral implant (ABG modular and nonmodular designs, Stryker, Mahwah, New Jersey).

opening clearing a path for flexible osteotomes. Sequential insertion of the osteotomes met resistance at an area of firm bone at the base of the ingrowth zone of the femoral stem. Continued trial of various osteotomes was unsuccessful at extraction and aborted secondary to concern of fracture. An extended trochanteric osteotomy was then performed. Once the implant was extracted, the proximal bone stock was examined and confirmed to be thin, as seen on radiographs. At this point, diaphyseal fixation seemed necessary and a Wagner SL stem (Zimmer, Warsaw, Indiana) was selected. The appropriate reamers were used and good fixation was achieved a trial implant. After trial reduction and range of motion, the real implant was placed and the trochanter was reduced to the diaphysis. A standard 5-hole trochanteric grip plate (Accord, Smith & Nephew, Memphis, Tennessee) was placed laterally and secured first with 2 cables under the lesser trochanter and then 3 additional cables around the diaphysis providing secure, solid fixation and reconstruction (**Fig. 9**).

Well-fixed stable short stem implants afford the possibility of safe and effective revision surgery with greater preservation of femoral bone and less-invasive technique.

Proximal-Distal Mismatch

The lack of a long distal stem in short stem femoral components also lends flexibility and adaptability with the broad range of proximal femoral morphology that exists.[22] The presence of proximal metaphyseal-distal diaphyseal mismatch in young, vigorous patients with robust, thick diaphyseal cortices and large cancellous metaphyses presents particular challenges to conventional-length uncemented implants (**Fig. 10**). Furthermore, avoiding proximal-distal mismatch in osteoporotic bone with disproportionately widened and weakened cortices lessens the risk of femoral perforation. Although those scenarios are common, cases of proximal femoral deformity are less common but equally challenging. In patients with excessively bowed femurs, deformed bone as a

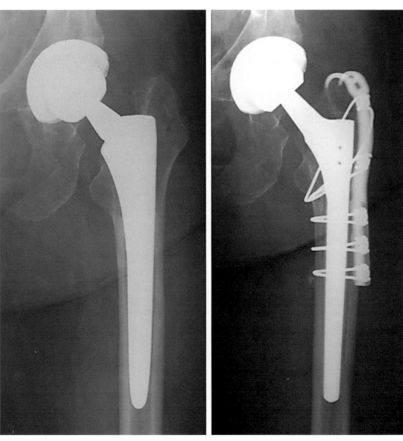

Fig. 9. (*Left*) Prerevision (Rejuvenate, Stryker, Mahwah, New Jersey) and (*right*) postrevision (Wagner SL, Zimmer, Warsaw, Indiana) radiographs of a conventional-length uncemented femoral implant.

A   **B**

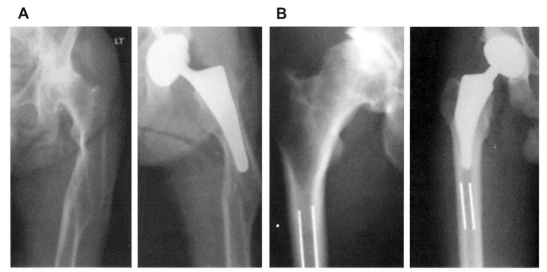

Fig. 10. Two types of proximal-distal mismatch treated with metaphyseal-engaging, short stem devices. (*A*) Proximal femoral fracture. (*B*) Wide metaphysis, narrow diaphysis in a young, robust male patient.

consequence of fracture or developmental abnormality short stem femoral implants may be able to provide adequate fixation while avoiding the area of deformity (see **Fig. 10**).

Use in Less-invasive Exposures

The smaller size of short stem implants lends itself to minimally invasive surgerical (MIS) approaches in THA. Molli and colleagues[34] found a lower complication rate with the use of short stem implants (0.4%) compared with conventional-length implants (3.1%) via a less-invasive direct lateral approach. In the short stem group, there was 1 femoral fracture. In the conventional-length stem group, there were 9 femoral fractures and 3 trochanteric avulsions. Lombardi and associates[45] found similar results with the use of the direct anterior approach for THA. Femoral fractures can be fixed intraoperatively with cerclage cables and lateral plates, but postoperative activity and function are impeded in the short term. MIS and less-invasive approaches can limit visualization of the subtrochanteric femoral shaft and may make safe insertion of longer stems more difficult than short stem implants.

CLINICAL AND RADIOGRAPHIC RESULTS OF SHORT STEM FEMORAL IMPLANTS

Short-term follow-up of anatomic uncemented short stem implants have been shown to provide pain relief, functional restoration, and stability similar to conventional uncemented designs (**Table 1**). The authors' center has recently published up to 7-year clinical and radiographic

follow-up of a CT-based custom short stem femoral implant. The femoral stem was made of titanium alloy with a hydroxyapatite coating on a titanium plasma spray in the proximal one-third to one-half of the stem (Biomet, Warsaw, Indiana) with an average stem length of 90 mm (range, 70–105 mm) (**Fig. 11**). HHSs averaged 55 (20–90) preoperatively and 96 (55–100) postoperatively. WOMAC scores averaged 51 (13–80) preoperatively and 3 (0–35) postoperatively. No cases of subsidence were observed and no revision surgeries have been performed. Bone remodeling was typified by endosteal condensation and cortical hypertrophy in Gruen zones 2, 3, 5, and 6.

This custom implant inspired the use of an off-the-shelf metaphyesal implant with a similar design. The authors prospectively followed 148 hips in 139 consecutive patients treated with an uncemented metaphyseal-engaging short (91–105 mm) stem that fit closely against the endosteal metaphyseal bone along the anterior metaphysis, medial calcar, posterior femoral neck, and metaphyseal flare at the bottom of the greater trochanter (Citation, Stryker, Mahwah, New Jersey) (see **Figs. 2**A and **6**C). At an average follow-up of 67 months, mean HHSs and WOMAC scores for the off-the-shelf cohort were 94 (range, 55–100) and 3.3 (range, 0–27), respectively. A subgroup of these patients was also evaluated to reveal stable fixation and comparable clinical outcomes in patients over the age of 70 years. Two-year follow-up of 60 patients (65 hips) 70 years and older (mean, 75 years; range, 70–86 years) with the Citation short stem revealed

Table 1
Summary of short uncemented femoral implants of various designs examined in cohorts of various ages

Study	Implant Design	Stem Fixation Type	N (Hips)	Average Postoperative HHS	Average Age (y)	Average Follow-up (y)	Stem Revisions for Aseptic Loosening
Patel et al,[49] 2012	Anatomic off-the-shelf short stem	Uncemented with hydroxyapatite	65	88	75	3	0 (0%)
Morrey et al,[29] 2000	Short stem with high valgus neck	Uncemented	20	98	N/A	2	1 (5%)
Pipino et al,[30] 2000	Anatomic femoral neck-sparing with collar	Uncemented	44	37% excellent, 45% good	62.5	13–17	0 (0%)
Santori & Santori,[31] 2010	Custom high-neck resection short stem	Uncemented with hydroxyapatite	129	95	51	8	0 (0%)
Morrey et al,[29] 2000	Double tapered short stem modular neck	Uncemented	159	90.4	51	6	3 (1.8%)
Morales de Cano et al,[35] 2013	Tapered short stem with elliptic-octagon cross-section	Uncemented with grit-blasted titanium	81	Merle d'Aubigné score: 16	65	1.3	0 (0%)
Molli et al,[34] 2012	Tapered flat-wedge short stem	Uncemented with porous plasma spray	269	83	63	2.3	0 (0%)
Ghera & Pavan,[46] 2009	Wedge femoral neck-sparing short stem	Uncemented with hydroxyapatite	50	91	70	1.7	0 (0%)
Lazovic & Zigan,[47] 2006	Modular femoral neck-sparing short stem	Uncemented with plasma Ca-P coating	55	92	48	0.5	0 (0%)
Rohrl et al,[48] 2006	Modular femoral neck-sparing short stem	Uncemented	26	93	54	2	0 (0%)
Patel et al,[36] 2013	Anatomic custom short stem	Uncemented with hydroxyapatite	69	96	56	5.5	0 (0%)

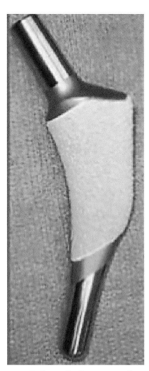

Fig. 11. Custom, CT-based, short stem femoral implant made of titanium alloy with a hydroxyapatite coating on a titanium plasma spray in the proximal one-third to one-half of the stem (Biomet, Warsaw, Indiana).

average HHSs of 88 (range, 70–100) and WOMAC scores of 6 (range, 0–43).

Another institution familiar with short stem femoral implants compared a large cohort of conventional-length femoral implants (Mallory-Head Porous, Biomet, Warsaw, Indiana) and short stem femoral implants (TaperLoc Microplasty, Biomet, Warsaw, Indiana). They found equivalent clinical and functional scores between 389 conventional-length stems and 269 short stems at average 29-month follow-up. Furthermore, they found a decreased complication rate (0.4%) in the short stem group compared with the conventional-length group (3.1%).

Santori and Santori reported reliable clinical and radiographic results in 129 custom-made uncemented high femoral neck resection short stem implants up to 8 years (**Fig. 12**). The indications for the use of this stem in this cohort were age of less than 60 years and good bone stock.

Although older generations of short stem femoral implants have longer follow-up (ie, Proxima [Depuy, Warsaw, IN] and Mayo Conservative Hip Prosthesis [Zimmer, Warsaw, IN]), newer generations lack long-term clinical and radiographic data.[29,30,41] One important difference in the 2 generations of implants is the surface coating. Initial

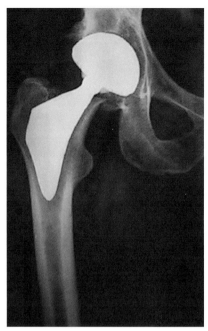

Fig. 12. Custom-made uncemented short stem femoral components (Stanmore Implants Worldwide, Elstree, United Kingdom, and Depuy International, Leeds, United Kingdom).

short stem implants were typically grit blasted with the extent and location varying significantly. Newer generations promote ingrowth with a porous coating and have osteoconductive stimulation via hydroxyapatite. This may explain the lower rate of subsidence in newer-generation short stem implants. Nevertheless, the success of older-generation implants and midterm success of newer-generation implants imply long-term clinical and functional success equivocal to conventional uncemented implants. Moreover, the benefits of soft tissue and bone preservation with short stem implants promote consideration of these implants. Increasing concerns regarding the use of metal-on-metal surface replacement arthroplasties are also stimulating interest in the development of reliable, safe, tissue-preserving short stem femoral implants as a possible alternative to surface replacements.

SUMMARY

In conclusion, uncemented femoral implants of various designs have proved to provide stable initial and long-term fixation in patients who undergo THA. Challenges in primary THA have led to the evolution of short stem designs. These challenges include proximal/metaphyseal and distal/diaphyseal mismatch; facilitation of less-invasive surgical exposures, especially the direct anterior approach; and bone preservation for potential revision surgery. The results of short stem implants with follow-up to 10 years strongly suggest that these implants will assume an increasingly important role in total hip arthroplasty.

REFERENCES

1. Berend KR, Lombardi AV, Mallory TH, et al. Cementless double-tapered total hip arthroplasty in patients 75 years of age and older. J Arthroplasty 2004;19(3): 288–95.

2. Berend ME, Smith A, Meding JB, et al. Long-term outcome and risk factors of proximal femoral fracture in uncemented and cemented total hip arthroplasty in 2551 hips. J Arthroplasty 2006; 21(6 Suppl 2):53–9.

3. Burt CF, Garvin KL, Otterberg ET, et al. A femoral component inserted without cement in total hip arthroplasty. A study of the Tri-Lock component with an average ten-year duration of follow-up. J Bone Joint Surg Am 1998;80(7):952–60.

4. Capello WN, D'Antonio JA, Jaffe WL, et al. Hydroxyapatite-coated femoral components: 15-year minimum followup. Clin Orthop Relat Res 2006;453: 75–80.

5. Rothman RH, Hozack WJ, Ranawat A, et al. Hydroxyapatite-coated femoral stems. A matched-pair analysis of coated and uncoated implants. J Bone Joint Surg Am 1996;78(3):319–24.

6. Meding JB, Galley MR, Ritter MA. High survival of uncemented proximally porous-coated titanium alloy femoral stems in osteoporotic bone. Clin Orthop Relat Res 2010;468(2):441–7.

7. Meding JB, Keating EM, Ritter MA, et al. Minimum ten-year follow-up of a straight-stemmed, plasma-sprayed, titanium-alloy, uncemented femoral component in primary total hip arthroplasty. J Bone Joint Surg Am 2004;86(1):92–7.

8. Muirhead-Allwood SK, Sandiford N, Skinner JA, et al. Uncemented custom computer-assisted design and manufacture of hydroxyapatite-coated femoral components: survival at 10 to 17 years. J Bone Joint Surg Br 2010;92(8):1079–84.

9. Albrektsson T, Branemark PI, Hansson HA, et al. Osseointegrated titanium implants. Requirements for ensuring a long-lasting, direct bone-to-implant anchorage in man. Acta Orthop Scand 1981;52(2): 155–70.

10. Aldinger PR, Breusch SJ, Lukoschek M, et al. A ten- to 15-year follow-up of the cementless spotorno stem. J Bone Joint Surg Br 2003;85(2):209–14.

11. Aldinger PR, Jung AW, Pritsch M, et al. Uncemented grit-blasted straight tapered titanium stems in patients younger than fifty-five years of age. Fifteen to twenty-year results. J Bone Joint Surg Am 2009; 91(6):1432–9.

12. Archibeck MJ, Berger RA, Jacobs JJ, et al. Second-generation cementless total hip arthroplasty. Eight to eleven-year results. J Bone Joint Surg Am 2001; 83(11):1666–73.

13. Berry DJ, Harmsen WS, Ilstrup D, et al. Survivorship of uncemented proximally porous-coated femoral components. Clin Orthop Relat Res 1995;(319): 168–77.

14. Bidar R, Kouyoumdjian P, Munini E, et al. Long-term results of the ABG-1 hydroxyapatite coated total hip arthroplasty: analysis of 111 cases with a minimum follow-up of 10 years. Orthop Traumatol Surg Res 2009;95(8):579–87.

15. Boden H, Salemyr M, Skoldenberg O, et al. Total hip arthroplasty with an uncemented hydroxyapatite-coated tapered titanium stem: results at a minimum of 10 years' follow-up in 104 hips. J Orthop Sci 2006; 11(2):175–9.

16. Bojescul JA, Xenos JS, Callaghan JJ, et al. Results of porous-coated anatomic total hip arthroplasty without cement at fifteen years: a concise follow-up of a previous report. J Bone Joint Surg Am 2003; 85(6):1079–83.

17. Bourne RB, Rorabeck CH. A critical look at cementless stems. Taper designs and when to use alternatives. Clin Orthop Relat Res 1998;(355): 212–23.

18. Bourne RB, Rorabeck CH, Patterson JJ, et al. Tapered titanium cementless total hip replacements: a 10- to 13-year followup study. Clin Orthop Relat Res 2001;(393):112–20.

19. Bugbee WD, Culpepper WJ II, Engh CA Jr, et al. Long-term clinical consequences of stress-shielding after total hip arthroplasty without cement. J Bone Joint Surg Am 1997;79(7):1007–12.

20. Baltopoulos P, Tsintzos C, Papadakou E, et al. Hydroxyapatite-coated total hip arthroplasty: the impact on thigh pain and arthroplasty survival. Acta Orthop Belg 2008;74(3):323–31.

21. Bauer TW, Geesink RC, Zimmerman R, et al. Hydroxyapatite-coated femoral stems. Histological analysis of components retrieved at autopsy. J Bone Joint Surg Am 1991;73(10):1439–52.

22. Noble PC, Alexander JW, Lindahl LJ, et al. The anatomic basis of femoral component design. Clin Orthop Relat Res 1988;(235):148–65.

23. Delaunay C, Bonnomet F, North J, et al. Grit-blasted titanium femoral stem in cementless primary total hip arthroplasty: a 5- to 10-year multicenter study. J Arthroplasty 2001;16(1):47–54.

24. Hofmann AA, Feign ME, Klauser W, et al. Cementless primary total hip arthroplasty with a tapered, proximally porous-coated titanium prosthesis: a 4- to 8-year retrospective review. J Arthroplasty 2000;15(7):833–9.

25. McTighe T, Stulberg SD, Keppler L, et al. A Classification System for Short Stem Uncemented Total Hip

Arthroplasty. Bone Joint Journal Orthopaedic Proceedings Supplement 2013;95(Suppl 15):260.

26. Freeman MA. Why resect the neck? J Bone Joint Surg Br 1986;68(3):346–9.

27. Pipino F, Calderale PM. Biodynamic total hip prosthesis. Ital J Orthop Traumatol 1987;13(3):289–97.

28. Whiteside LA, White SE, McCarthy DS. Effect of neck resection on torsional stability of cementless total hip replacement. Am J Orthop (Belle Mead NJ) 1995;24(10):766–70.

29. Morrey BF, Adams RA, Kessler M. A conservative femoral replacement for total hip arthroplasty. A prospective study. J Bone Joint Surg Br 2000;82(7):952–8.

30. Pipino F, Molfetta L, Grandizio M. Preservation of the femoral neck in hip arthroplasty: results of a 13- to 17-year follow-up. J Orthop Traumatol 2000;1(1):31–9.

31. Santori FS, Santori N. Mid-term results of a custom-made short proximal loading femoral component. J Bone Joint Surg Br 2010;92(9):1231–7.

32. Leali A, Fetto J. Promising mid-term results of total hip arthroplasties using an uncemented lateral-flare hip prosthesis: a clinical and radiographic study. Int Orthop 2007;31(6):845–9.

33. Walker P, Culligan S, Hua J, et al. The effect of a lateral flare feature on uncemented hip stems. Hip International 1999;9(2):71–80.

34. Molli RG, Lombardi AV Jr, Berend KR, et al. A short tapered stem reduces intraoperative complications in primary total hip arthroplasty. Clin Orthop Relat Res 2012;470(2):450–61.

35. Morales de Cano JJ, Gordo C, Illobre JM. Early clinical results of a new conservative hip stem. Eur J Orthop Surg Traumatol 2013. [Epub ahead of print].

36. Patel RM, Lo WM, Cayo MA, et al. Stable, Dependable Fixation of Short-stem Femoral Implants at 5 Years. Orthopedics 2013;36(3):e301–7.

37. Reimeringer M, Nuno N, Desmarais-Trepanier C, et al. The influence of uncemented femoral stem length and design on its primary stability: a finite element analysis. Comput Methods Biomech Biomed Engin 2012. [Epub ahead of print].

38. Pilliar RM, Lee JM, Maniatopoulos C. Observations on the effect of movement on bone ingrowth into porous-surfaced implants. Clin Orthop Relat Res 1986;(208):108–13.

39. Schmidutz F, Graf T, Mazoochian F, et al. Migration analysis of a metaphyseal anchored short-stem hip prosthesis. Acta Orthop 2012;83(4):360–5.

40. Arno S, Fetto J, Nguyen NQ, et al. Evaluation of femoral strains with cementless proximal-fill femoral implants of varied stem length. Clin Biomech (Bristol, Avon) 2012;27(7):680–5.

41. Chen HH, Morrey BF, An KN, et al. Bone remodeling characteristics of a short-stemmed total hip replacement. J Arthroplasty 2009;24(6):945–50.

42. Weinans H, Huiskes R, Grootenboer HJ. Effects of material properties of femoral hip components on bone remodeling. J Orthop Res 1992;10(6):845–53.

43. Sychterz CJ, Claus AM, Engh CA. What we have learned about long-term cementless fixation from autopsy retrievals. Clin Orthop Relat Res 2002;(405):79–91.

44. Patel AR, Patel RM, Thomas D, et al. Caveat Emptor: adverse inflammatory soft-tissue reactions in total hip arthroplasty with modular femoral neck implantsa report of two cases. J Bone Joint Surgery Case Connector 2012;2(4):e80.1–6.

45. Lombardi AV Jr, Berend KR, Adams JB. A short stem solution: through small portals. Orthopedics 2009;32(9).

46. Ghera S, Pavan L. The DePuy Proxima hip: a short stem for total hip arthroplasty. Early experience and technical considerations. Hip international: the journal of clinical and experimental research on hip pathology and therapy 2009;19(3):215.

47. Lazovic D, Zigan R. Navigation of short-stem implants. Orthopedics 2006;29(10):125–9.

48. Röhrl S, Li MG, Pedersen E, et al. Migration pattern of a short femoral neck preserving stem. Clinical orthopaedics and related research 2006;448:73–8.

49. Patel RM, Smith MC, Woodward CC, et al. Stable fixation of short-stem femoral implants in patients 70 years and older. Clin Orthop Relat Res 2012;470(2):442–9.

Trauma

Preface
Trauma

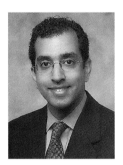

Saqib Rehman, MD
Editor

The current issue of *Orthopedic Clinics of North America* has three topics dedicated to orthopedic trauma, which we trust you will find timely and potentially useful in your clinical practice. Intramedullary nailing of tibia fractures typically presents a technical challenge when treating proximal injuries. Malreductions are frequent without the use of blocking screws, certain reduction techniques, and alternative positioning. Drs Mir and Stinner have provided their expertise in treating these particular injuries in their review/technique article. Peripheral nerve injuries are a dreaded complication of surgical treatment of fractures and other orthopedic conditions. These can occur preoperatively, intraoperatively, or postoperatively due to compression, traction, ischemia, or a combination of mechanisms. Dr Plastaras and colleagues have tackled this topic in the form of two articles: upper extremity and lower extremity peripheral nerve

traction injuries. Finally, Dr Sullivan and colleagues have written on the complex topic of spondylopelvic dissociation. Whereas unilateral sacral fractures are typically part of the injury pattern seen in many pelvic ring injuries and are well-understood, U-shaped and related patterns can be missed, are treated with unfamiliar methods, and, if not properly treated, can lead to complete loss of sacral nerve function. I hope that you and our readers enjoy this particular issue.

Saqib Rehman, MD
Department of Orthopaedic Surgery
Temple University Hospital
3401 North Broad Street
Philadelphia, PA 19140, USA

E-mail address:
Saqib.rehman@tuhs.temple.edu

orthopedic.theclinics.com

Techniques for Intramedullary Nailing of Proximal Tibia Fractures

Daniel J. Stinner, MD, Hassan Mir, MD*

KEYWORDS

- Proximal tibia fracture • Extra-articular • Suprapatellar nailing • Retropatellar nailing
- Semiextended nailing • Blocking screws

KEY POINTS

- Despite poor early results with intramedullary nailing of extra-articular proximal tibia fractures, improvements in surgical technique and implant design modifications have resulted in more acceptable outcomes.
- Prevention of the commonly encountered apex anterior and/or valgus deformities remains a challenge when treating these injuries.
- It is necessary for the surgeon to recognize that prevention of apex anterior and/or valgus deformities presents a constant challenge and it is their responsibility to know how to neutralize these forces.
- Surgeons should be comfortable using a variety of the reduction techniques presented to minimize fracture malalignment.

INTRODUCTION

Proximal tibia fractures have presented a treatment challenge for orthopedic surgeons. Soft tissue concerns with open plating techniques resulted in the increased use of either percutaneous plating methods or intramedullary nail (IMN) fixation, which has the added benefit of being a load-sharing device to allow early weight bearing. Malalignment was common with early nailing techniques and implant designs as demonstrated by several series published during the 1990s.[1,2] In a radiographic analysis of 133 tibia fractures treated with IMN fixation, Freedman and Johnson[2] reported that 7 (58%) of the 12 proximal tibia fractures were malaligned, compared with an overall malalignment rate of all tibia fractures of 12% in the study. This experience was shared by Lang and colleagues[1] who evaluated the results of 32 extra-articular proximal third tibia fractures treated with an IMN. At final follow-up, 27 (84%) of 32 fractures were malaligned more than 5° in the sagittal or coronal plane. As a result, the authors stated that they have limited their use of IMN for proximal third fractures.

The common deformity seen in proximal third tibia fractures is an apex anterior and/or valgus deformity. There are two main factors that complicate reduction of extra-articular proximal tibial fractures when treated with closed IMN: deforming forces of the proximal tibia (mainly extension of the proximal segment caused by pull of the extensor mechanism, but also forces from pull of the

Funding Sources: None.

Conflict of Interest: The opinions or assertions contained herein are the private views of the authors and are not to be construed as official or as reflecting the views of the Department of the Army or the Department of Defense (D.J. Stinner). Paid consultant for Smith and Nephew (H. Mir).

Division of Orthopaedic Trauma, Vanderbilt Orthopaedic Institute, Vanderbilt Medical Center, Medical Center East, Suite 4200, Nashville, TN 37232, USA

* Corresponding author.

E-mail address: Hassan.mir@vanderbilt.edu

hamstrings and iliotibial band in different patterns); and the spaciousness of the intramedullary canal proximal to the metaphyseal flare.[3–5]

IMN fixation offers several significant advantages over other treatment methods, such as plate fixation, because patients can be allowed to weight bear earlier and the surgery can be performed without making large skin incisions over a potentially compromised soft tissue envelope. The clinical benefits of treating these injuries with IMNs led surgeons to make implant design modifications and improve surgical techniques to yield the results we have today with malalignment rates of less than 8% in several recent series.[6,7]

IMPLANT DESIGN

Some reasons for failure in treatment, defined by malalignment or loss of fixation, can be in part attributed to early implant design. Early generation tibial nails had a proximal sagittal bend (Herzog curve) that was larger than currently available nails, and/or had a bend that extended distal to the fracture site. Both of these design characteristics contribute to what Henley and coworkers[8] referred to as the "wedge effect," which occurs as the nail is seated and impinges on the posterior cortex of the distal segment accentuating an apex anterior deformity because of the effective widening of the nail above the bend and posterior force on the distal segment to match the nail shape.

Additional reasons for early fixation failure in these fractures have been attributed to use of a single proximal interlocking bolt, or use of the dynamic interlocking mode. Both Henley and coworkers[8] and Laflamme[9] demonstrated the problems associated with limited fixation in the proximal segment, and implant modifications to include additional oblique/multiplanar interlocking bolt options have minimized loss of fracture reduction.

Further modifications to IMN design have included the addition of angular stable locking screws that thread into the nail. Although they seem to offer additional stability, especially in osteoporotic bone, when compared with conventional implants (nonthreaded locking holes) using a biomechanical proximal tibia fracture model they offered no extra benefit.[10]

NAIL STARTING POINT

The starting point should be just medial to the lateral tibia spine on the anteroposterior (AP) fluoroscopic image (ensure appropriate rotation using the fibular bisector line or the "twin peaks" view) and just anterior to the articular surface on the lateral fluoroscopic image ("flat plateau").

Obtaining the correct starting point is important for nailing proximal tibia fractures for two reasons. First, just as in standard nailing for tibia fractures, the surgeon should avoid damage to the intra-articular structures. Tornetta and colleagues[11] have detailed the safe zone for tibial nailing, which is 9.1 ± 5 mm lateral to midline of the plateau and 3 mm lateral to the center of the tubercle. The width averaged between 22.9 and 12.6 mm. A follow-up study was performed to identify the fluoroscopic images that correlate with the appropriate safe zone. Kirschner wires were placed in cadaveric knees under direct visualization of the safe zone, and then radiographs were obtained that demonstrated that the safe zone is just medial to the lateral tibial spine on the AP and just anterior to the articular surface on the lateral image. There was some variance on the AP, but no variance on the lateral image.[12]

A recent study confirmed the importance of obtaining appropriate intraoperative fluoroscopic images, because a slight external rotation of the proximal tibia when obtaining fluoroscopic images of the starting point can result in a misleading medial entry point, which may accentuate a valgus deformity. The authors of this study used the fibular bisector line (overlap of the lateral border of the tibia bisecting the fibula head) as a reliable intraoperative fluoroscopic confirmation of appropriate rotation because the entry point using this image was always either ideal or less than 5 mm lateral to the ideal entry point, but never medial.[13] Because of the potential valgus deformity obtained with intramedullary nailing of proximal tibia fractures, avoidance of a medial starting point is paramount.

An alternative method for ensuring appropriate rotation on intraoperative fluoroscopic images is use of the twin peaks AP view and flat plateau lateral view.[14] A cadaveric study demonstrated excellent intraobserver and interobserver reliability with use of this technique compared with use of the fibular bisection line on the AP view and perfectly aligned femoral condyles on the lateral view, allowing for accurate identification of the starting point. The twin peaks AP view simply obtains the sharpest profile of the tibial spines and the flat plateau lateral view lines up the posterior aspect of the femoral condyles and then adducts the limb to line up the medial and lateral tibial plateaus (**Figs. 1** and **2**).

NAILING TECHNIQUES
Nailing in Flexion

- Hyperflexion permits accurate guidewire placement and alignment in sagittal plane.

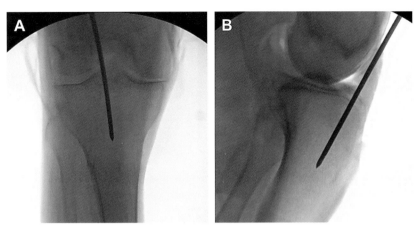

Fig. 1. Fluoroscopic images demonstrating use of the fibular bisector line on the AP image (*A*) and the lateral of the knee using the overlapping outline of the femoral condyles (*B*).

- The incision can be medial, through, or lateral to the patellar tendon to facilitate accurate pin placement.
- Ensure trajectory of guidewire or awl is correct on intraoperative fluoroscopy before reaming the proximal tibia.
- Fracture must be reduced before canal preparation (reaming) and implant placement.
- Place locking bolts with limb in extension (the position of reduction).

The traditional method of nailing tibia fractures, regardless of location of the fracture, has been to nail in flexion. Hyperflexion of the knee allows accurate placement and alignment of the guidewire in the sagittal plane, nearly parallel to the anterior cortex. The incision is most commonly medial to the patellar tendon, but can be midline or even lateral to the tendon in certain cases to facilitate accurate pin placement and minimize interference from the extensor mechanism.[15] After preparation of the entry portal, it is important to extend the knee for reduction, canal preparation, and placement of the interlocking bolts.[4] This balances the deforming forces on the proximal tibia in the sagittal plane to assist in maintenance of reduction. However, it must be emphasized that the fracture should always be reduced before or while reaming and nailing, because simply extending the leg without using proper technique throughout the procedure does not compensate for the resultant deformity with nail passage. This point likely led to modifications to the implant system and surgical technique to accommodate nailing in the semi-extended position, making it easier to keep the fracture reduced while reaming and during passage of the IMN.

Nailing in Semiextended Position

- Limit flexion to approximately 15° to neutralize the force of the extensor mechanism on the

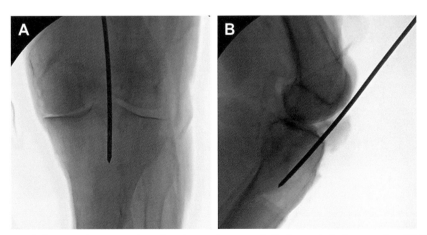

Fig. 2. Fluoroscopic images demonstrating the alternative use of "twin peaks" view on the AP (*A*) and "flat plateau" view on the lateral (*B*) fluoroscopic images.

proximal tibia leading to an apex anterior deformity, and to relax the tissues allowing for easier instrumentation in proper alignment. The slight flexion allows access to the proximal tibia to obtain the correct starting point.

  ○ This can be done with small radiolucent bump or triangle behind the knee, which allows for slight flexion. In addition, the use of an elevated radiolucent leg ramp elevates the injured extremity above the contralateral leg, making intraoperative fluoroscopy easier (**Figs. 3** and **4**).

- The approach can be made medial or lateral to the patellar tendon depending on which way it is easier to subluxate the patella.
- Trochlear groove used as an alignment guide for instrumentation.
- Ensure trajectory of guidewire or awl is correct on intraoperative fluoroscopy before reaming the proximal tibia.
- Fracture must be reduced before canal preparation (reaming) and implant placement.

Tornetta and Collins[16] were one of the first to describe nailing proximal tibia fractures in the semiextended position with the use of an arthrotomy. Of 25 patients with proximal tibia fractures treated with IMNs by this technique, 19 had anatomic alignment in the sagittal plane, and none had greater than 5° malalignment in the sagittal plane. Two of the 25 had coronal plane deformities greater than 5°. In a prospective study, Vidyadhara and Sharath[17] had a 16% malunion rate in 7 of 45 patients with proximal tibia fractures treated with intramedullary nailing in the semiextended position, three in valgus and four apex anterior greater than 5°. Variations of this semiextended technique have been reported with the use of extra-articular approaches.[18,19]

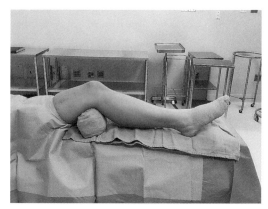

Fig. 4. A bump placed under the knee may be used to aid in obtaining optimal knee flexion to obtain the correct starting point.

Suprapatellar Nailing

- Similar amount of knee flexion (15°) required as in semiextended to neutralize the force of the extensor mechanism on the proximal tibia leading to an apex anterior deformity. The slight flexion allows access to the proximal tibia to obtain the correct starting point.

  ○ An elevated radiolucent leg ramp is used to elevate the injured extremity above the contralateral leg, making intraoperative fluoroscopy easier.

  ○ A small radiolucent bump is required under the knee to obtain appropriate amount of knee flexion.

- Skin incision is approximately 2 cm in length, starting 2 cm above patella and extending proximally (**Fig. 5**).
- Quadriceps tendon is well visualized, with deep incision through its midsubstance, stopping 5 mm above superior patellar pole.

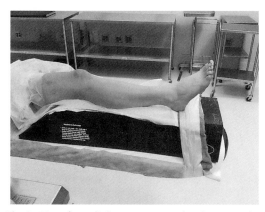

Fig. 3. Use of a radiolucent ramp under the operative extremity aids in achieving slight knee flexion while elevating the operative extremity above the contralateral limb, making intraoperative fluoroscopy easier.

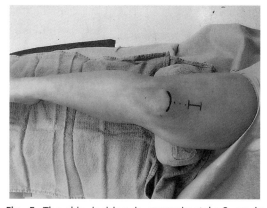

Fig. 5. The skin incision is approximately 2 cm in length, starting 2 cm above the superior pole of the patella (outlined with the *dark curvilinear line*), mid axis.

- Finger palpation of the patellofemoral space to assess if adequate room for the trocar to be placed.
  - If more space is needed (ie, trocar does not fit or is very tight), determine which way the patella subluxates more freely and cut 1 to 2 cm of the patellar retinaculum medially or laterally to allow subluxation of the patella, leaving a cuff for later extensor mechanism repair.
- Ensure trocar/cannula placed down to tibia to ensure that the femoral condyles and patella are not damaged when instrumenting/reaming, or by the cannula edge with sliding.
- Systems may allow securing the cannula to the distal femur with a wire, which ensures cannula does not back out during the procedure putting condyles and patella at risk of damage by the reamer and cannula edge. If system does not have this feature, always ensure cannula pushed down at all times.
- Trochlear groove used as an alignment guide for instrumentation.
- Ensure trajectory of guidewire is correct on intraoperative fluoroscopy before reaming the proximal tibia.
- Fracture must be reduced before canal preparation (reaming) and implant placement.
- Systems may allow nail to be passed through cannula. Ensure that system does allow if desired, and size nail chosen will fit through the cannula because certain systems' cannulas can only accommodate certain size nails.
- At the conclusion of the procedure, thoroughly irrigate knee and assess patellofemoral joint.

More recently, the suprapatellar or retropatellar approach has gained popularity because of the relative ease with which the appropriate starting point can be identified using the trochlear groove as a guide, and the ability to keep the leg in one position throughout reaming and nail insertion (**Figs. 6** and **7**). Even with this technique, the optimum amount of knee flexion remains somewhere around 15°, which allows for a more accurate placement of the initial guidewire in the safe zone at the appropriate insertion angle.[16,20]

One of the initial concerns with suprapatellar nailing was caused by the thought that the contact pressures of the implants or instruments would be high enough to cause damage to the surrounding cartilage. In a study evaluating contact pressures using a modern nailing system that has a suprapatellar cannula, an increase in the mean pressure on the cartilaginous surfaces was found for suprapatellar compared with infrapatellar technique. However, suprapatellar technique had a mean of 1.84 MPa (range, 1.09–2.95 MPa) on the patella and 2.13 MPa (range, 1.10–2.86 MPa) on the femoral condyles, which is much lower than that which can impair the structural integrity of the cartilage with a single impact (>25 Mpa) and nearly half the pressures required to induce chondrocyte apoptosis with sustained loads (4.5 Mpa) in immature bovine cartilage.[21]

Additionally, a recent cadaveric study demonstrated that another benefit to the retropatellar technique when compared with parapatellar nailing is a significant decrease in the damage to intra-articular structures, with a similarly sized resultant entry hole and anterior cortical damage in the proximal tibia.[22] Whether this has any clinical significance has yet to be demonstrated.

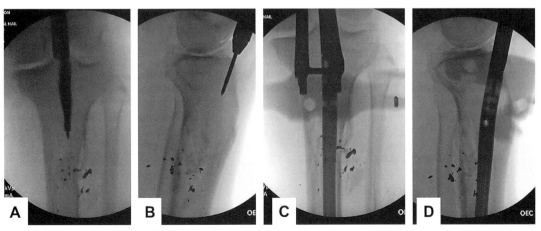

Fig. 6. Intraoperative AP (*A*) and lateral (*B*) fluoroscopic images demonstrating the ease with which the correct starting point can be found and the ease with which alignment is maintained without much, if any, manipulation of the extremity during passage of the nail (*C, D*).

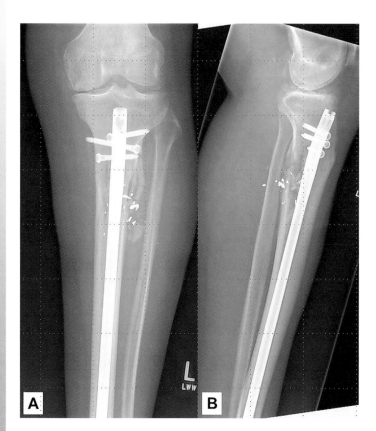

Fig. 7. Postoperative AP (*A*) and lateral (*B*) radiographs demonstrating maintenance of alignment in a case using the suprapatellar technique.

REDUCTION TECHNIQUES
Clamp-assisted Reduction

- Ensure safe passage of clamps when placed percutaneously, especially along the posterior border of the proximal tibia.
- Attention to soft tissue impingement is paramount with percutaneous clamp placement; if the tissues are compressed, alternative wider periarticular clamps may be helpful.
- Caution should be exercised because clamps may loosen with canal instrumentation, vibrations from reaming, and passage of the nail.

Although not commonly described for proximal tibia fractures, the use of percutaneous clamps can be extremely effective in obtaining and maintaining reduction while reaming and during passage of the nail (**Figs. 8** and **9**). The use of percutaneous clamps has resulted in good outcomes in comminuted tibial shaft fractures and distal third tibia fractures.[23,24] It is often easier to place clamps in open fractures because one can directly visualize clamp placement; however, they can also be effectively used in closed injuries through stab incisions. Caution should be exercised when placing percutaneous clamps to reduce the flexion deformity seen in proximal tibia fractures by ensuring that the clamp remains in contact with the bone all the way around the posterior aspect of the proximal tibia. Attention to soft tissue impingement is paramount with percutaneous clamp placement because narrow pointed reduction forceps pinching the skin may cause tissue necrosis if left in place for even short amounts of time. If the tissues are compressed, alternative wider periarticular clamps may be helpful.

Blocking/Poller Screws

- Ideal time for blocking screw placement is before reaming and placing the nail.
  - Can also be placed later in the procedure to
    - Correct deformity with nail removal and rereaming.
    - To enhance construct stability in metaphyseal fracture with poor bone quality or comminution.
- If placing before reaming, the authors recommend using larger screws or the systems interlocking bolts, because smaller screws (≤3.5 mm) may bend or break under load caused by weakening if a portion of the screw

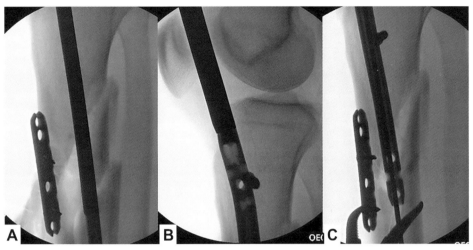

Fig. 8. Intraoperative lateral fluoroscopic view demonstrating apex anterior deformity with a segmental proximal tibia fracture after nail passage (using suprapatellar technique), even with a temporary plate used to assist with alignment of the proximal fracture (*A*). Addition of a blocking screw and clamp-assisted reduction resulted in improved alignment in the coronal plane (*B, C*).

is reamed. Do not use a drill bit as a blocking pin because they can be brittle and break. Can also consider a 3.2-mm (more flexible) or larger Steinman pin, which can be removed after locking the nail (the "stealth" blocking screw).

- Several nailing systems have targeters for placing blocking screws.
- Beware of fracture propagation and watch carefully under fluoroscopy. Consider placing the blocking screws at least 1 cm away from fracture to minimize risk.

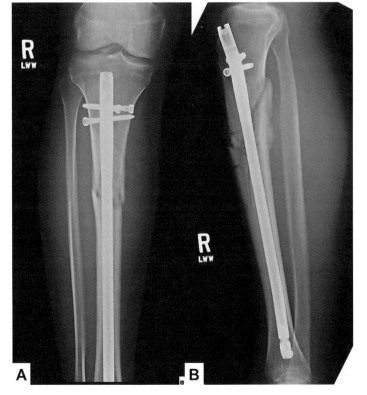

Fig. 9. Postoperative AP (*A*) and lateral (*B*) radiographs of the patient shown in **Fig. 8**, demonstrating appropriate final alignment. Note that the temporary plate shown in **Fig. 8** was removed after locking the nail.

Because of the cavernous proximal tibia and the typical deformity associated with proximal tibia fractures, blocking screws, also referred to as Poller screws, have been used to decrease the effective size of the proximal tibia, thus controlling the IMN path in the proximal tibia and helping to mitigate potential malalignment.[25] Blocking screws are always placed on the concavity of the deformity. For proximal tibia fractures, which have a typical apex anterior and valgus deformity, the blocking screws can be placed lateral and/or posterior to the nail in the proximal segment. **Figs. 10–16** demonstrate simulated and clinical application of blocking screws. Krettek and colleagues[26] also demonstrated that, in addition to improving and maintaining alignment, blocking screws offer a biomechanical advantage when used in the treatment of proximal tibia fractures because they increase the overall bone-implant-construct stability. Therefore, consideration may be given in certain cases (osteoporosis, comminution) to adding Poller screws to enhance construct stability, even if they were not required to obtain alignment.

Good success in obtaining and maintaining alignment using blocking screws has been demonstrated in several clinical series. Ricci and coworkers[27] reported on 12 consecutive patients and only had one postoperative malalignment of 6° of valgus that progressed to 10° at final follow-up; however, in this case, no blocking screws were used. In all other cases, the fractures healed with no clinical malalignment. The use of blocking screws can generate significant forces so the surgeon should beware of fracture propagation and watch carefully under fluoroscopy during each step. Consideration should be given to placing the blocking screws at least 1 cm away from fracture to minimize risk, because fracture propagation can lead to either construct instability with metadiaphyseal extension or articular incongruity with proximal fracture extension.

Plate-assisted Reduction

- Use a 3.5-mm dynamic compression plate (DCP) or limited contact dynamic compression plate (LC-DCP), five- or six-hole plate with minimum of two screws on both sides of the fracture. Less stout implants or points of fixation can lead to loosening during nail implantation and subsequent loss of reduction.
- Use unicortical screws or place bicortical outside the projected path of the nail.
- Remove plate after locking the nail, or leave in place, with possible exchange of unicortical screws for bicortical screws.
- Although this technique is often reserved for open fractures, it can be considered for closed fractures when alignment cannot be obtained or maintained with other techniques.

One of the difficulties with proximal tibia fractures is not just obtaining a reduction, but maintaining it

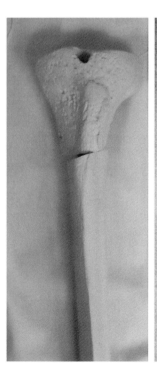 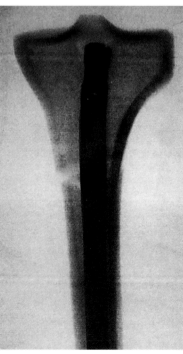

Fig. 10. The typical valgus deformity present after nail insertion for a proximal tibia fracture is shown.

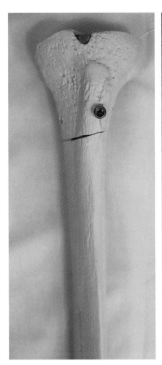
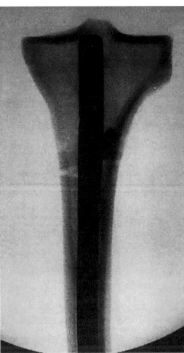

Fig. 11. The valgus deformity seen in **Fig. 10** has been corrected with placement of a lateral blocking screw in the proximal segment.

while reaming and placing the implant. A provisional plate can be added to assist in obtaining and maintain reduction, more commonly done in open fractures because the tibia has already been exposed for debridement, but also in select closed fractures when other closed and percutaneous methods are unsuccessful. Several studies have reported good results using this technique.

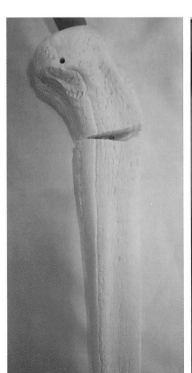
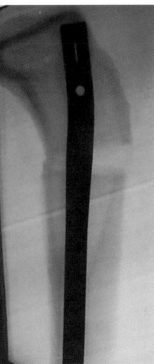

Fig. 12. The typical apex anterior (procurvatum) deformity present after nail insertion for a proximal tibia fracture is shown.

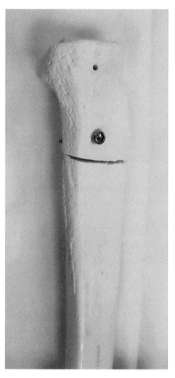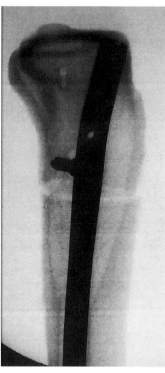

Fig. 13. The apex anterior (procurvatum) deformity seen in Fig. 12 has been corrected with placement of a posterior blocking screw in the proximal segment.

Because of the amount of force that can be transmitted when placing an IMN, the authors recommend using a 3.5-mm DCP or LC-DCP plate. Using a less stout plate (ie, one-third tubular plate) can result in loss of reduction and bending of the plate during nail passage (personal experience). Typically, only a five- or six-hole plate is all that is necessary. Screws are either placed

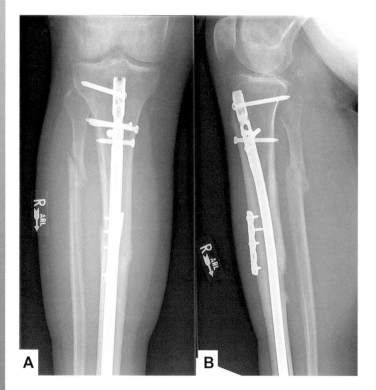

Fig. 14. (A, B) Radiographs demonstrating a healed tibia fracture with appropriate alignment achieved with use of blocking screws, both in the sagittal and coronal plane, in addition to the use of plate-assisted reduction, which was left in place.

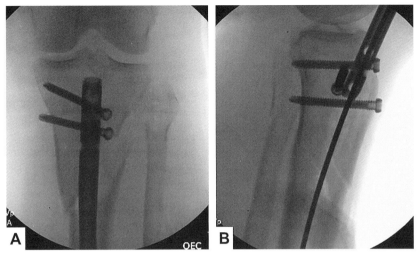

Fig. 15. Fluoroscopic image demonstrating typical valgus deformity after locking the nail proximally. Of note, the patient had a segmental tibia fracture and the proximal fracture was not recognized until fluoroscopic imaging obtained to check proximal locking bolt lengths (*A*). The nail was subsequently removed and blocking screws added, two in the sagittal plane and one in the coronal plane, followed by rereaming and nail placement (*B*).

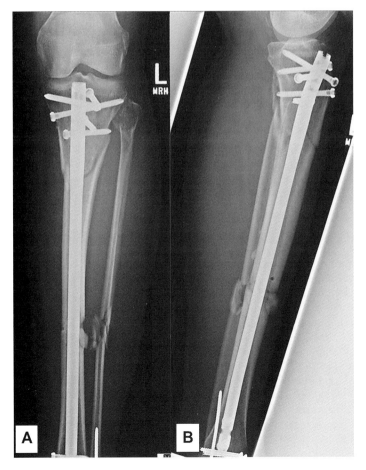

Fig. 16. Postoperative AP (*A*) and lateral (*B*) radiographs demonstrate improved final alignment of the patient shown in **Fig. 15** after the addition of blocking screws to aid in reduction of the proximal tibia fracture.

unicortically or bicortically directed around the anticipated nail path. The plating should be performed with no iatrogenic periosteal stripping. After the nail is passed and interlocking bolts placed, the plate can be removed, left in place with unicortical screws, or left in place with screws exchanged for bicortical screws around the nail (see **Figs. 8**, **9**, and **14**).[6,7,28]

Dunbar and colleagues[7] performed provisional plating in 31 fractures, removing the plate after the nail was locked. In 18 patients the alignment remained anatomic and in the other 13, there was less than 3° of malalignment. Nork and colleagues[6] used plate-assisted reduction in 13 proximal quartile extra-articular tibia fractures. Three plates were temporary and removed after placing the IMN, and in the other 10 cases, the unicortical screws were exchanged for bicortical screws after the locking screws were placed. In this series, other techniques were also used to include the use of a femoral distractor, with acceptable alignment (<5° malalignment) obtained in 34 (92%) of 37 fractures, two with 5° malalignment and one with 7° malalignment.

Universal Distractor

- A medially based universal distractor can be used to correct multiplanar deformity.
- Consider placing the proximal Schanz pin in a manner that would act as a blocking screw to prevent an apex anterior deformity.
- Ensure placement of distal Schanz pin is out of (or distal to) the anticipated trajectory of the nail.

In the study by Nork and colleagues[6] describing their outcomes on proximal quartile tibia fractures treated with an IMN, a medial distractor was placed in 68% of cases. It can be applied medially to counteract the valgus deformity by "dialing in" the coronal alignment. Although no blocking screws were using in this study, the proximal Schanz pin for the distractor was placed in a manner to behave like a blocking screw. In that study, 34 of 37 fractures had less than 5° angular deformity, 2 had 5° (coronal), 1 had 7° (coronal).

Wysocki and colleagues[29] modified this technique using a two-pin fixator construct. The authors described using 2- to 5-mm centrally threaded transfixion pins connected to carbon fiber rods medially and laterally creating a form of traveling traction that can aid in fracture reduction. The authors also used "strategic placement of a bump" to aid in correction of sagittal plane deformity. Using this technique on 15 proximal and distal tibia fractures, the authors reported 14 with angular deformity less than 5°.

SUMMARY

Despite poor early results with intramedullary nailing of extra-articular proximal tibia fractures, improvements in surgical technique and implant design modifications have resulted in more acceptable outcomes. However, prevention of the commonly encountered apex anterior and/or valgus deformities remains a challenge when treating these injuries. It is necessary for the surgeon to recognize this and know how to neutralize these forces. Surgeons should be comfortable using a variety of the reduction techniques presented to minimize fracture malalignment.

REFERENCES

1. Lang GJ, Cohen BE, Bosse MJ, et al. Proximal third tibial shaft fractures. Should they be nailed? Clin Orthop Relat Res 1995;(315):64–74.
2. Freedman EL, Johnson EE. Radiographic analysis of tibial fracture malalignment following intramedullary nailing. Clin Orthop Relat Res 1995;(315):25–33.
3. Hak DJ. Intramedullary nailing of proximal third tibial fractures: techniques to improve reduction. Orthopedics 2011;34:532–5.
4. Buehler KC, Green J, Woll TS, et al. A technique for intramedullary nailing of proximal third tibia fractures. J Orthop Trauma 1997;11:218–23.
5. Hiesterman TG, Shafiq BX, Cole PA. Intramedullary nailing of extra-articular proximal tibia fractures. J Am Acad Orthop Surg 2011;19:690–700.
6. Nork SE, Barei DP, Schildhauer TA, et al. Intramedullary nailing of proximal quarter tibial fractures. J Orthop Trauma 2006;20:523–8.
7. Dunbar RP, Nork SE, Barei DP, et al. Provisional plating of type III open tibia fractures prior to intramedullary nailing. J Orthop Trauma 2005;19: 412–4.
8. Henley MB, Meier M, Tencer AF. Influences of some design parameters on the biomechanics of the unreamed tibial intramedullary nail. J Orthop Trauma 1993;7:311–9.
9. Laflamme GY, Heimlich D, Stephen D, et al. Proximal tibial fracture stability with intramedullary nail fixation using oblique interlocking screws. J Orthop Trauma 2003;17:496–502.
10. Thelen S, Betsch M, Grassmann JP, et al. Angle stable locking nails versus conventionally locked intramedullary nails in proximal tibial shaft fractures: a biomechanical study. Arch Orthop Trauma Surg 2012;132:57–63.
11. Tornetta P III, Riina J, Geller J, et al. Intraarticular anatomic risks of tibial nailing. J Orthop Trauma 1999;13:247–51.
12. McConnell T, Tornetta P III, Tilzey J, et al. Tibial portal placement: the radiographic correlate of

the anatomic safe zone. J Orthop Trauma 2001;15: 207–9.

13. Walker RM, Zdero R, McKee MD, et al. Ideal tibial intramedullary nail insertion point varies with tibial rotation. J Orthop Trauma 2011;25:726–30.

14. Bible JE, Choxi AA, Dhulipala S, et al. Tibia-based referencing for standard proximal tibial radiographs during intramedullary nailing. Am J Orthop, in press.

15. Althausen PL, Neiman R, Finkemeier CG, et al. Incision placement for intramedullary tibial nailing: an anatomic study. J Orthop Trauma 2002;16:687–90.

16. Tornetta P III, Collins E. Semiextended position of intramedullary nailing of the proximal tibia. Clin Orthop Relat Res 1996;(328):185–9.

17. Vidyadhara S, Sharath KR. Prospective study of the clinico-radiological outcome of interlocked nailing in proximal third tibial shaft fractures. Injury 2006;37: 536–42.

18. Kubiak EN, Widmer BJ, Horwitz DS. Extra-articular technique for semiextended tibial nailing. J Orthop Trauma 2010;24:704–8.

19. Morandi M, Banka T, Gaiarsa GP, et al. Intramedullary nailing of tibial fractures: review of surgical techniques and description of a percutaneous lateral suprapatellar approach. Orthopedics 2010; 33:172–9.

20. Eastman J, Tseng S, Lo E, et al. Retropatellar technique for intramedullary nailing of proximal tibia fractures: a cadaveric assessment. J Orthop Trauma 2010;24:672–6.

21. Gelbke MK, Coombs D, Powell S, et al. Suprapatellar versus infra-patellar intramedullary nail insertion of the tibia: a cadaveric model for comparison of patellofemoral contact pressures and forces. J Orthop Trauma 2010;24:665–71.

22. Bible JE, Choxi AA, Dhulipala S, et al. Quantification of anterior cortical bone removal and intermeniscal ligament damage at the tibial nail entry zone using parapatellar and retropatellar approaches. J Orthop Trauma 2013;27(8):437–41.

23. Kim KC, Lee JK, Hwang DS, et al. Percutaneous reduction during intramedullary nailing in comminuted tibial shaft fractures. Orthopedics 2008;31: 556–9.

24. Forman JM, Urruela AM, Egol KA. The percutaneous use of a pointed reduction clamp during intramedullary nailing of distal third tibial shaft fractures. Acta Orthop Belg 2001;77:7.

25. Krettek C, Stephan C, Schandelmaier P, et al. The use of Poller screws as blocking screws in stabilising tibial fractures treated with small diameter intramedullary nails. J Bone Joint Surg Br 1999;81: 963–8.

26. Krettek C, Miclau T, Schandelmaier P, et al. The mechanical effect of blocking screws ("Poller screws") in stabilizing tibia fractures with short proximal or distal fragments after insertion of small-diameter intramedullary nails. J Orthop Trauma 1999;13:550–3.

27. Ricci WM, O'Boyle M, Borrelli J, et al. Fractures of the proximal third of the tibial shaft treated with intramedullary nails and blocking screws. J Orthop Trauma 2001;15:264–70.

28. Kim KC, Lee JK, Hwang DS, et al. Provisional unicortical plating with reamed intramedullary nailing in segmental tibial fractures involving the high proximal metaphysis. Orthopedics 2007;30:189–92.

29. Wysocki RW, Kapotas JS, Virkus WW. Intramedullary nailing of proximal and distal one-third tibial shaft fractures with intraoperative two-pin external fixation. J Trauma 2009;66:1135–9.

Perioperative Upper Extremity Peripheral Nerve Traction Injuries

Christopher T. Plastaras, MD[a],*, Akhil Chhatre, MD[b],
Ashot S. Kotcharian, MD[a]

KEYWORDS

- Perioperative • Upper extremity • Peripheral nerve • Traction injuries

KEY POINTS

- Perioperative peripheral nerve traction injury is a poorly understood complication, with multiple etiopathologic considerations.
- Presentation may vary along the spectrum of sensory and motor nerve injury.
- Nerve injury can occur along any part of the path traversed, with bias of predisposing factors, like medical comorbidity and female gender.
- Potential nerve and plexus injury surrounding shoulder and elbow surgery are examined.

INTRODUCTION

The occurrence of perioperative peripheral nerve traction injuries (PPNTI) during upper and lower extremity orthopedic procedures such as joint replacements is an uncommon and unpleasant complication. PPNTI are regrettable complications of surgery, believed to arise from stretch or compression of vulnerable peripheral nerves secondary to retraction as well as patient limb positioning. PPNTI remains a poorly understood complication, with an incidence that is largely unknown and difficult to establish. Part of the reason for this difficulty is that in a lot of cases the cause of a perioperative nerve injury is unknown.[1] Another reason why it is difficult to establish an incidence for PPNTI is that a definition of a traction injury is not always consistent between investigators. Depending on the investigator, the definition may vary from positioning or retraction, and if compression injury is included, it may be a stretch injury caused by compression or a combination of some of these. Therefore, in most studies, the incidence given for a perioperative nerve injury is all inclusive, and

few studies[2] give a PPNTI-specific incidence. Other common mechanisms of surgery-related nerve injuries besides traction include compression, entrapment, direct trauma (eg, crushing or laceration injuries), and indirect trauma (eg, secondary to hematoma formation).[3]

PATHOPHYSIOLOGY

PPNTI is a type of nerve injury in which inappropriate placement of a noncompliant external object, such as retraction, may create an external pressure on the nerve, producing nerve ischemia and injury. Traction nerve injuries can be acute or chronic. An abrupt external force resulting in the immediate loss of function from the consequential structural changes of the neural tissue causes the acute traction injury. With a chronic traction injury, the nerve is stretched so slowly that considerable deformation of neural tissue occurs before the signs and symptoms appear.

The amount of stretch that a nerve tolerates depends on whether the nerve is freely mobile in supple soft tissue or whether it is bound down by

[a] Department of Physical Medicine and Rehabilitation, University of Pennsylvania Perelman School of Medicine, 1800 Lombard Street, Philadelphia, PA 19146, USA; [b] Department of Neurological Surgery, Johns Hopkins University, 600 N. Wolfe Street, Baltimore, MD, USA
* Corresponding author.
E-mail address: Christopher.Plastaras@uphs.upenn.edu

Orthop Clin N Am 45 (2014) 47–53
http://dx.doi.org/10.1016/j.ocl.2013.09.006

osseous prominences, fascia, or scar. In Lundborg and Rydevik's study of the sciatic nerve of rabbits,[4] histologic changes were found after lengthening of nerves by 4% to 11%, nerve microcirculation was impaired after 8% stretch and stopped after 15% stretch, and there was conduction failure with 25% lengthening. The rupture of axon fibers precedes the failure of fascicles and may occur with stretch of as little as 4% to 6%.[5] A more recent functional and mechanical evaluation of nerve stretch injury found the minimum threshold for nerve stretch before functional deficit to be between 5% and 10%.[6] The theory is that stretching causes narrowing of both the extraneural and intraneural microvasculature and results in impaired blood flow. Lundborg and Rydevik also studied the temporal effects of ischemia and showed that restoration of blood flow after 2 hours of tourniquet-induced ischemia resulted in complete recovery of nerve function, with no edema in the epineurium or endoneurium. The development of endoneurial edema seems to be the hallmark of irreversible nerve injury.

Four major factors that increase the probability of mechanical disruption are increased load because of compression or stretch, increased rate of loading, increased duration of loading, and uneven application of load to tissues.[7] Clinical experience and the Laplace law (tension is proportional to the pressure and radius of a cylindrical structure) show that large-diameter axons are more susceptible to damage than smaller fibers. Animal models have shown that peripheral nerves are especially sensitive to compression injury.[8] If peripheral nerves are sensitive to compression, then it is possible that some traction injuries may not be secondary to stretch and tension but possibly caused by markedly increased compression from a near osseous or prosthetic prominence while the nerve is stretched. Yet another mechanism is from development of postoperative scar tissue, which puts tension on a nerve, resulting in chronic traction. Reinnervation rates vary depending on the location or severity of the injury and the length to the target tissue (muscle or sensory organ). Reinnervation can occur between 3 and 4 mm/d in nerve injuries when the endoneurial sheath is intact; however, after nerve suture, if reinnervation occurs, the rate decreases to 0.5 to 1 mm/d.[9]

CLASSIFICATION OF PERIPHERAL NERVE INJURIES

The most widely accepted classifications of nerve injuries are those described by Seddon (neuropraxia, axonotmesis, and neurotmesis)

and by Sunderland (grade 1–5 nerve injuries). According to the Seddon classification,[10] nerve injuries can be classified into 3 categories: neuropraxia (mild: focal demyelination after focal injury; axon intact), axonotemesis (moderate: axonal loss; nerve sheath intact), and neurotmesis (severe: axonal loss and disruption of nerve sheath).

CLINICAL PRESENTATION OF PERIPHERAL NERVE TRACTION INJURIES

Just as any peripheral nerve injury, PPNTI may lead to sensory or motor deficits. Sensory deficit can present as anesthesia, paresthesia, hypoesthesia, hyperesthesia, and pain in the areas supplied by the affected nerves. Motor deficits can include paresis or even paralysis of the affected muscles. Nerve-specific clinical presentations are discussed later.

GENERAL PREDISPOSING FACTORS TO PPNTI

Medical comorbidities that result in microvascular changes, such as hypertension, diabetes mellitus, and smoking, may render these patients to be more susceptible to PPNTI.[3,11,12] It is also reported that rheumatoid arthropathy of the knee is a common predisposition for peroneal palsy after total knee arthroplasty.[13,14] Preexisting peripheral neuropathies also predispose to a PPNTI.[15] Other predisposing factors include anatomic sites of susceptibility (discussed in greater detail later) and anesthesia factors (general and epidural anesthesia are associated with a higher incidence of PPNTI). Perioperative factors such as hypovolemia, dehydration, hypotension, hypoxia, electrolyte disturbances, and hypothermia have also been implicated in the development of PPNTI. At least in studies of total hip arthroplasties, women are more at risk for peripheral nerve injury than men.[16–19] A possible explanation is that compared with men, women have smaller bodies, with shorter limbs, and therefore shorter nerves as well. Because nerve stretch injury begins at about 4% to 11% elongation from the original length, individuals with shorter nerves need less stretch.[20]

What is important to understand when discussing general and specific predisposing factors is that although there are several preoperative, perioperative, and postoperative factors that have been reported to be significant for the development of PPNTI, no single entity has been consistently shown in all studies to be significant, and some patients without any known risk factor still develop PPNTI.

PERIPHERAL NERVE TRACTION INJURIES OF THE UPPER LIMB
Status After Shoulder Surgery

The nerves in the immediate vicinity of the operative field include the brachial plexus and its branches (axillary, musculocutaneous, suprascapular, subscapular). The incidence of such nerve injuries varies with the procedure, the approach used, and anatomic variation, as well as with the skill and experience of the surgeon. The reported incidence is 1% to 2% in patients undergoing rotator cuff surgery, 1% to 8% in patients undergoing surgery for anterior instability, and 1% to 4% in patients undergoing arthroplasty.[21] However, because injury is usually identified clinically only and because of the difficulty of examining a shoulder postoperatively, true incidence may be even higher.

Brachial plexus injury (C5-T1)
Incidence The incidence of brachial plexus injury is believed to range from 0.2% to 0.6%.[3] Some studies have looked to intraoperative monitoring of nerves to obtain a better idea of incidence of nerve traction injury and predisposing factors. In a study by Nagda and colleagues[22] of 30 patients in whom the brachial plexus nerves were continuously monitored during shoulder arthroplasty, 17 (56.7%) had 30 nerve alerts (episodes of nerve dysfunction) during surgery. None of these 30 nerve alerts returned to baseline with retractor removal alone. After repositioning of the arm into a neutral position, 23 (76.7%) of the 30 alerts returned to baseline. In those alerts that did not return to baseline, 4 of 7 (57.1%) had positive postoperative electromyography results.

Predisposing factors Given its superficial nature and its proximity to several mobile bony structures, the brachial plexus is susceptible to injury. Other predisposing factors include running between 2 fixed points (intervertebral foramen and the axillary sheath), and its course through a limited space between the clavicle and first rib, which also make the plexus susceptible to injury. There also seems to be some increased risk of neurologic complications in patients with history of previous open shoulder surgery on the involved extremity.[22] Whether this situation is caused by poor compliance and stretching of scar tissue, resulting in inability of nerves to slide within planes and an increase in local traction, or if it is caused by the need to be placed in more extreme positions for longer periods to obtain an appropriate surgical view, is unknown.

Mechanism of injury Compression and traction against the clavicle may occur during retraction or in the lateral decubitus position with compression against the thorax and humeral head. Arm abduction and external rotation with posterior shoulder displacement cause considerable stretch on the upper brachial plexus roots. In the intraoperative nerve monitoring study by Nagda and colleagues, the nerve events were triggered during portions of the procedure when the surgical extremity was placed into extreme external rotation, extension, and either abduction or adduction. When the amount of external rotation and extension was decreased, most nerve compromise was reduced or eliminated, lending support to the theory that injury was likely secondary to traction. Nagda and colleagues' findings are supported by biomechanical data from Kwaan and Rappaport.[23] These investigators used strain gauge testing to delineate that an arm placed in 90° of abduction, external rotation, and slight extension produced traction on the brachial plexus.

Clinical presentation If the C5-6 nerve roots are affected with involvement of the musculocutaneous, axillary, and suprascapular nerves, the arm is medially rotated, adducted, and pronated, classically described as the waiter's tip position. If C8-T1 roots are involved, the small muscles of the hand are then involved, resulting in a claw hand and numbness in the ulnar distribution.

Prevention and treatment Proper positioning and avoiding excessive shoulder abduction, extension, and external rotation should help decrease chance of nerve injury. Some advocate for intraoperative monitoring to avoid nerve injury, and 1 study has shown transcranial electrical motor-evoked potentials to be sensitive indicators of impending injury to the brachial plexus or peripheral nerves during shoulder arthroplasty and also proximal humeral fracture repairs.[24] Should a brachial plexus nerve injury be diagnosed, it is important early on to support the involved upper extremity in order to avoid further traction.

Axillary nerve injury (C5-6)
Axillary nerve injury has been documented during various procedures, including shoulder arthroplasty, the Bristow transfer, and Bankart repair.[12]

Incidence Varies from 1% to 7% of cases.[10]

Predisposing factors The axillary nerve is susceptible to injury at the quadrilateral space, near the anteroinferior border of the glenohumeral capsule and the inferior border of the subscapularis muscle. The nerve is particularly susceptible to stretch after it curves around the posterolateral surface of the humerus deep to the deltoid and divides into anterior and posterior branches, where it is tethered posteriorly, as a result of the overlying muscle, making it susceptible to stretch.[25]

Mechanism of injury The mechanism of injury is compression against the neck of the humerus and posterior stretch at the tethered zone, described earlier.

Clinical presentation The presenting complaint is usually arm fatigue with overhead activity or throwing. Examination shows weak lateral abduction and external rotation of the arm. There may be associated paresthesias of the lateral and posterior upper arm.

Prevention and treatment Preventive measures that should be used during dissection include careful nerve identification and retractor use. In the lateral approach, the axillary nerve can be protected and displaced away from the operative field with adduction and external rotation of the arm.[12,21] Externally rotating the humerus not only helps expose the area of surgical interest but also helps reduce tension on the axillary nerve. In the posterior approach, it is recommended to stay above the teres minor because of the axillary nerve as well as the posterior circumflex humeral artery, both running in the quadrilateral space below the teres minor. Using an appropriately flat retractor helps minimize traumatic traction.

In arthroscopic shoulder procedures, incorrect trochar direction and portal placement can endanger nerves. Care must be used during dissection or portal placement in this region. For posterior portal placement, the posterolateral corner of the acromion is used as a landmark for the skin incision, aiming approximately 2 cm inferior and 1 cm medial to it. Once the portal is in, the trochar should be directed toward the coracoid. The axillary nerve can be at risk for injury if the portal is made too low. If the portal is made too medial, the suprascapular nerve may be in danger. The anterior portal can be established using an inside-out technique using a Wissenger rod or by puncture of the anterior skin under direct vision from the posterior portal.[21]

If a permanent axillary nerve injury occurs, successful management may include free sural nerve grafting at 3 to 6 months postoperatively, an option that is reported to result in successful recovery of strength to grade 4 of 5.[26] Another option is transferring the nerve innervating the medial head of the triceps to the anterior axillary nerve.[12]

Musculocutaneous nerve injury (C5-7)

Incidence PPNTI of the musculocutaneous nerve is rare and there are no incidences mentioned in the literature and only 1 case report.[27]

Predisposing factors Because proximally, the musculocutaneous nerve may bifurcate and has an unpredictable entry point into the coracobrachialis muscle, it is particularly vulnerable to injury in its proximal course, where it lies on the subscapularis muscle.[21] Any surgical procedures involving the anterior aspect of the shoulder therefore risk injuring the musculocutaneous nerve, such as the modified Bristow procedure (for shoulder instability) or shoulder arthroscopy (because of joint distension, excessive traction, and extravasation of fluid).[12,21]

Mechanism of injury During the Bristow transfer, the transfer of the conjoined tendon may cause tenting and increased tension on the musculocutaneous nerve branch after successful transfer.[5] During arthroscopic shoulder procedures, the musculocutaneous nerve is at risk if the anterior portal is placed too medial.

Clinical presentation Weakness of flexion of the elbow and numbness along the lateral border of the forearm are seen if there is involvement of the musculocutaneous nerve.

Prevention and treatment In the lateral approach of shoulder surgery, the musculocutaneous nerve can be protected by avoiding vigorous retraction of the coracobrachialis, short head of biceps conjoint tendon, and any dissection medial to coracobrachialis.[21]

Given the possibility of anatomic variation, it is recommended that before tendon transfer, the musculocutaneous nerve is identified, and if the anatomic variation is identified, then the tendon transfer should be aborted or a complete neurolysis should be completed before tendon transfer.

Status After Elbow Surgery

Elbow arthroscopy and reconstruction of the ulnar collateral ligament of the elbow have been associated with neurologic injury to the radial, median, and ulnar nerves and their various branches in up to 14% and 31% of cases, respectively.[12]

Radial nerve injury (C5-T1)

Incidence Radial injury incidence of 4% to 12% is reported for humeral shaft fracture operative treatments, depending on approach used.[28]

Predisposing factors Arising from the posterior cord, the radial nerve becomes vulnerable at 2 sites: as it tracks along the spiral groove of the humerus, where it is in direct contact with the periosteum (a distance of about 6 cm), and also at the point where it pierces and is tethered by the lateral intermuscular septum.[29]

Mechanism of injury Common perioperative reasons cited for radial nerve injury include compression against a patient screen or an arm board positioned at an incorrect height, creating a step. Other commonly cited reasons include tourniquets and arterial pressure cuffs. In elbow arthroscopy, the radial nerve is at particular risk during placement of an anterolateral portal, which is most commonly located 5 to 10 mm posterolateral to the radial nerve.[30] A high risk of injury to the radial nerve has also been noted in arthroscopic contracture release.[31]

Clinical presentation Clinical presentation typically includes wrist drop and numbness along the posterior surface of the lower part of the arm, posterior surface of the forearm, and the lateral 3 and a half digits on the dorsal side, as well as a small area on the dorsum of the hand.

Prevention and treatment Taking care in proper positioning so that the arm is not compressed against a rigid structure is important in prevention of injury. In arthroscopic procedures, recommendations for preventing nerve injury include 90° of flexion to help displace vital structures in the antecubital fossa away from the portal placement site; careful placement of the anterolateral portal relative to local anatomic landmarks; cautious debridement in the posterior compartment during contracture release.[12]

Median nerve injury (C5-T1)

Incidence The median nerve is most commonly injured during carpal tunnel release, with an incidence in about 0.1% of cases.[32] It is not known what fraction of those cases of median nerve injury were PPNTI.

Predisposing factors The nerve is susceptible to compression and stretch at the carpal tunnel. Variant anatomy of the median nerve may increase risk of iatrogenic injury.[33]

Mechanism of injury When an unpadded pronated arm is left hanging off the table, the median nerve may become compressed and stretched as it traverses the upper arm on the table edge.[34] Hyperextension of the elbow may place the median nerve at risk for injury.[35] Compression or stretch of the nerve may occur during insertion of the endoscopic cannula or with hand positioning.[36]

Clinical presentation Median nerve injury results in paresthesia along the palmar aspect of the lateral 3 and a half fingers. Motor manifestations include weakness of abduction and opposition of the thumb, weak wrist flexion, and the forearm being kept in supination. The muscles of the thenar eminence become wasted, and the hand appears flattened.

Prevention and treatment Careful limb positioning and padding, avoiding hyperextension of the elbow, and being mindful of the limb during the operation so as not to lean on it and exacerbate any compression or stretch are all important in preventing PPNTI. If postoperative median nerve palsy is identified, successful management has included exploration or sural nerve grafting, or repair with epineural sutures.[37]

Ulnar nerve injury (C8-T1)

Incidence The incidence of postoperative ulnar neuropathy has been reported between 0% and 51%,[38] and it is frequently reported to be the most common perioperative nerve injury. As many as 1 in 200 adult surgical patients are affected, and it seems that men are more vulnerable.[3,28] Two more recent studies have reported incidences of 20%[39] and 16%,[40] respectively. Again, these studies do not go on to stratify type of nerve injury acquired.

Predisposing factors Ulnar nerve injury seems to be caused by its superficial nature and closeness to the medial condyle. Because the nerve passes through the ulnar groove at the elbow, it is prone to several types of compressive injuries. It is possible that the ulnar nerve and its blood supply may be compromised by internal compression caused by the coronoid tubercle of the ulna. This bony prominence is at least 50% larger in men, consistent with the greater susceptibility to perioperative ulnar nerve damage seen in men.[3] It is also possible that in humeral fracture repair procedures, the type of fracture may be a risk factor for developing PPNTI. A study by Wiggers and colleagues[40] concluded that patients with columnar fractures might be at higher risk for the development of postoperative ulnar neuropathy than patients with capitellum and trochlea fractures. The investigators believed the increased risk to be likely because of more transposition involved in columnar fracture repairs, as well as the additional handling of the ulnar nerve that occurred with reduction of a columnar fracture and application of a medial plate.

Mechanism of injury Direct pressure on the ulnar groove in the elbow and prolonged forearm flexion are cited as the most common causes of injury.[3,28] Extreme flexion of the elbow (>90°) tightens the arcuate ligament and shrinks the cubital tunnel, increasing the risk of nerve compression in the tunnel. With sustained elbow flexion, an elongation of 5 to 14 mm of the nerve has been reported.[41] In repairs of supracondylar fractures of the humerus, it is widely accepted that medial pinning can damage the ulnar nerve not only by direct injury during insertion but also with elbow movement after insertion or by constricting the cubital tunnel.[42] It is possible that postoperative scarring may limit the inherent laxity of the ulnar nerve around the elbow, which protects it from traction and compression injury caused by elbow flexion, and can result in chronic traction injury.[43]

Clinical presentations Ulnar nerve injury is usually characterized by tingling or numbness along the little finger and weakness of fifth digit abduction, adduction, or both. Examination of the hand shows hyperextension of the metacarpophalangeal joints and flexion at the distal and the proximal interphalangeal joints of the ring and the little finger (ulnar claw).

Prevention and treatment Chances of nerve stretch or traction injury can be reduced with particular care in performing an elbow arthroscopy, especially when there has been previous trauma, surgery, or a congenital anomaly, because tethered or displaced nerves may render them vulnerable to injury.[44] Surgical treatment of ulnar nerve injury may include neurolysis or transposition, or sural nerve intercalary grafting in severe cases.[44]

NOTE: Please see following article entitled, "Perioperative Lower Extremity Peripheral Nerve Traction Injuries."

REFERENCES

1. Schmalzried TP, Amstutz HC, Dorey FJ. Nerve palsy associated with total hip replacement. J Bone Joint Surg Am 1991;73A:1074–80.
2. Telleria JJ, Safran MR, Gardi JN, et al. Risk of sciatic nerve traction injury during hip arthroscopy–is it the amount or duration? J Bone Joint Surg Am 2012;22:2025–32.
3. Lalkhen AG, Bhatia K. Perioperative peripheral nerve injuries. Cont Educ Anaesth Crit Care Pain 2012;12(1):38–42.
4. Lundborg G, Rydevik B. Effects of stretching the tibial nerve of the rabbit: a preliminary study of the intraneural circulation and the barrier function of the perineurium. J Bone Joint Surg Br 1973;55:390–401.
5. Bodine SC, Lieber RL. Peripheral nerve physiology, anatomy, and pathology. In: Simon SR, editor. Orthopaedic basic science. Rosemont (IL): American Academy of Orthopaedic Surgeons; 1994. p. 325–96.
6. Rickett T, Connel S, Bastijanic J, et al. Functional and mechanical evaluation of nerve stretch injury. J Med Syst 2011;35:787–93.
7. DeHart MM, Riley LH. Nerve injuries in total hip arthroplasty. J Am Acad Orthop Surg 1999;7:101–11.
8. De Luca CJ, Bloom LJ, Gilmore LD. Compression induced damage on in situ severed and intact nerves. Orthopedics 1987;10:777–84.
9. Sunderlund S. Nerve injuries and their repair. Edinburgh (Scotland): Churchill Livingstone; 1991.
10. Seddon HJ. Three types of nerve injuries. Brain 1943;66:237–88.
11. Welch MB, Brummett CM, Welch TD, et al. Perioperative peripheral nerve injuries. Anesthesiology 2009;111:490–7.
12. Maak TG, Osei D, Delos D, et al. Peripheral nerve injuries in sports-related surgery: presentation, evaluation, and management. J Bone Joint Surg Am 2012;94. e121(1–10).
13. Schinsky MF, Macaulay W, Parks ML, et al. Nerve injury after primary total knee arthroplasty. J Arthroplasty 2001;16:1048–54.
14. Knutson K, Leden I, Sturfelt G, et al. Nerve palsy after knee arthroplasty in patients with rheumatoid arthritis. Scand J Rheumatol 1983;12(3):201.
15. Horlocker TT, Cabanela ME, Wedel DJ. Does postoperative epidural analgesia increase the risk of peroneal nerve palsy after total knee arthroplasty? Anesth Analg 1994;79:495.
16. Nercessian OA, Macaulay W, Stinchfield FE. Peripheral neuropathies following total hip arthroplasty. J Arthroplasty 1994;9:645–51.
17. Johanson NA, Pellicci PM, Tsairis P, et al. Nerve injury in total hip arthroplasty. Clin Orthop Relat Res 1983;(179):214–22.
18. Solheim LF, Hagen R. Femoral and sciatic neuropathies after total hip arthroplasty. Acta Orthop Scand 1980;51(3):531–4.
19. Edwards BN, Tullos HS, Noble PC. Contributory factors and etiology of sciatic nerve palsy in total hip arthroplasty. Clin Orthop Relat Res 1987;(218):136–41.
20. Lewallen DG. Instructional course lectures, the American Academy of Orthopaedic Surgeons–neurovascular injury associated with hip arthroplasty. J Bone Joint Surg Am 1997;79:1870–80.
21. Rashid A, Abdul-Jabar H, Lam F. Nerve injury associated with shoulder surgery. Curr Orthop 2008;22:284–8.
22. Nagda SH, Rogers KJ, Sestokas AK, et al. Peripheral nerve function during shoulder arthroplasty

using intraoperative nerve monitoring. J Shoulder Elbow Surg 2007;16:2S–8S.

23. Kwaan JH, Rappaport I. Postoperative brachial plexus palsy: a study on the mechanism. Arch Surg 1970;101:612–5.

24. Warrender WJ, Oppenheimer S, Abboud JA. Nerve monitoring during proximal humeral fracture fixation: what have we learned? Clin Orthop Relat Res 2011; 469:2631–7.

25. Lee S, Saetia K, Saha S, et al. Axillary nerve injury associated with sports. Neurosurg Focus 2011;5: 1–7.

26. Yoneda M, Hayashida K, Wakitani S, et al. Bankart procedure augmented by coracoid transfer for contact athletes with traumatic anterior shoulder instability. Am J Sports Med 1999;27(1):21–6.

27. Ma H, Van Heest A, Glisson C, et al. Musculocutaneous nerve entrapment. Am J Sports Med 2009;37: 2467–9.

28. Zhang J, Moore AE, Stringer MD. Iatrogenic upper limb nerve injuries: a systematic review. ANZ J Surg 2011;81:227–36.

29. Carlan D, Pratt J, Patterson JM, et al. The radial nerve in the brachium: an anatomic study in human cadavers. J Hand Surg Am 2007;32:1177–82.

30. Kelly EW, Morrey BF, O'Driscoll SW. Complications of elbow arthroscopy. J Bone Joint Surg Am 2001; 83A(1):25–34.

31. Jones GS, Savoie FH 3rd. Arthroscopic capsular release of flexion contractures (arthrofibrosis) of the elbow. Arthroscopy 1993;9(3):277–83.

32. Benson L, Bare A, Nagle D, et al. Complications of endoscopic and open carpal tunnel release. Arthroscopy 2006;22:919–24.

33. Kretschmer T, Antoniadis G, Richter HP, et al. Avoiding iatrogenic nerve injury in endoscopic carpal tunnel release. Neurosurg Clin N Am 2009;20:65–71.

34. Winfree CJ, Kline DG. Intraoperative positioning nerve injuries. Surg Neurol 2005;63:5–18.

35. American Society of Anesthesiologists. Practice advisory for the prevention of perioperative peripheral neuropathies: a report by the American Society of Anesthesiologists Task Force on Prevention of Perioperative Peripheral Neuropathies. Anesthesiology 2000;92:1168–82.

36. Uchiyama S, Yasutomi T, Fukuzawa T, et al. Median nerve damage during two-portal endoscopic carpal tunnel release. Clin Neurophysiol 2004; 115:59–63.

37. Haapaniemi T, Berggren M, Adolfsson L. Complete transection of the median and radial nerves during arthroscopic release of post-traumatic elbow contracture. Arthroscopy 1999;15(7):784–7.

38. Robinson CM, Hill RM, Jacobs N, et al. Adult distal humeral metaphyseal fractures: epidemiology and results of treatment. J Orthop Trauma 2003;17: 38–47.

39. McKee MD, Veillette CJ, Hall JA, et al. A multicenter, prospective, randomized, controlled trial of open reduction–internal fixation versus total elbow arthroplasty for displaced intra-articular distal humeral fractures in elderly patients. J Shoulder Elbow Surg 2009;18:3–12.

40. Wiggers JK, Brower KM, Helmerhorst GT, et al. Predictors of diagnosis of ulnar neuropathy after surgically treated distal humerus fractures. J Hand Surg 2012;37A:1168–72.

41. Grewal R, Varitimidis SE, Vardakas DG, et al. Ulnar nerve elongation and excursion in the cubital tunnel after decompression and anterior transposition. J Hand Surg 2000;25B:457–60.

42. Rose RE, Phillips W. Iatrogenic ulnar neuropathies post-pinning of displaced supracondylar humerus fractures in children. West Indian Med J 2002;51: 17–20.

43. Novak CB, Mehdian H, von Schroeder HP. Laxity of the ulnar nerve during elbow flexion and extension. J Hand Surg 2012;37A:1163–7.

44. Gay DM, Raphael BS, Weiland AJ. Revision arthroscopic contracture displaced release in the elbow resulting in an ulnar nerve transection. J Bone Joint Surg Am 2010;92:1246–9.

Perioperative Lower Extremity Peripheral Nerve Traction Injuries

Christopher T. Plastaras, MD[a],*, Akhil Chhatre, MD[b], Ashot S. Kotcharian, MD[a]

KEYWORDS

- Perioperative • Lower extremity • Peripheral nerve traction injuries • Knee • Hip

KEY POINTS

- Perioperative peripheral nerve traction injury is a poorly understood known complication with multiple etiopathologic considerations.
- Presentation may vary along the spectrum of sensory and motor nerve injury.
- Nerve injury can occur along any part of the path traversed with bias of predisposing factors like medical comorbidity and female gender.
- Nerve conduction and electromyogram (EMG) studies are invaluable for determining the presence of nerve injury, localization, completeness, recovery, and prognostication.
- The authors examine potential nerve and plexus injury surrounding hip and knee surgery.
- Diagnosis is established with thorough history and physical examination, along with the aid of testing modalities, such as magnetic resonance imaging/ultrasound and diagnostic testing, such as EMG/nerve conduction studies.
- Careful assessment of patients, planned procedure, and risk factors are key to prevention.

NOTE: Please see preceding article entitled, "Perioperative Upper Extremity Peripheral Nerve Traction Injuries."

PERIPHERAL NERVE TRACTION INJURIES OF THE LOWER LIMB
Following Hip Surgery

Nerve injuries related to hip surgery may be the most-studied neurologic complication of joint surgery. The incidence of nerve damage following total hip arthroplasty (THA) varies from 0.09% to 7.6%, with incidences after primary THAs lower and after THA revision on the higher end.[1–15] Regarding hip arthroscopy, the incidence of nerve injury is comparable; one aggregation of the results of 30 studies found an 1.7% prevalence.[2] The exact cause of these postoperative peripheral nerve injuries are unknown 50% to 60% of the time.[1,14,16] Overall, most nerve palsies after THA have not been explored, with the assumption being that they are secondary to stretch injuries and would have a poor prognosis with exploration.

Farrell and colleagues[16] looked specifically for motor nerve palsy in 27,000 cases of THA and found the incidence to be 0.17%. In a review of 3126 consecutive total hip replacements, the incidence of nerve injury in hip arthroplasty was 1.7% overall, 1.3% when looking at primary hip replacements, and as high as 3.6% in hip revisions.[1] The same study also reported a much higher incidence for nerve injury in hip replacements for congenital

a Department of Physical Medicine and Rehabilitation, University of Pennsylvania Perelman School of Medicine, 1800 Lombard Street, Philadelphia, PA 19146, USA; b Department of Physical Medicine and Rehabilitation, Johns Hopkins University, 600 N. Wolfe Street, Baltimore, MD, USA
* Corresponding author.
E-mail address: Christopher.Plastaras@uphs.upenn.edu

Orthop Clin N Am 45 (2014) 55–63
http://dx.doi.org/10.1016/j.ocl.2013.09.005
0030-5898/14/$ – see front matter © 2014 Elsevier Inc. All rights reserved.

hip dislocations and the developmental dysplasia of the hip (5.2%). Again the researchers do not differentiate the type of nerve injury that make up this category, admitting that the cause was unknown in up to 57% of cases who had a peripheral nerve injury. They do attribute 13 cases to be secondary to tension caused by the limb lengthening involved in some of the hip replacements. Considering only these cases of neuropathy after hip replacement, the incidence of peripheral nerve traction injuries (PPNTI) would then be only 0.4%.

These numbers show that hip revisions, congenital dislocations/dysplasia, and leg lengthening are 3 risk factors for nerve injury. Other studies have come to the same conclusions.[11,12] Another risk factor that seems specific for hip arthroplasty is female sex.[14,17–19] The surgical approach used in THA may also be a risk factor. Farrell's results showed that the risk of nerve injury was significantly higher in patients operated on through a posterior approach than it was in those treated with an anterolateral or transtrochanteric approach.[16]

The sciatic nerve accounts for more than 80% of hip surgery–associated PPNTI, most of which is the peroneal division, with an isolated injury to the tibial portion being rare.[1] The next most commonly injured are the pudendal and femoral nerves.[20] Typically, the reported ratio of pudendal to sciatic nerve injury is approximately 1:3 with the patient in the lateral position and 2:1 with the patient in the supine position.[2] PPNTI of the superior and inferior gluteal as well as the obturator nerves are even more rare.

Sciatic nerve injury (L4–S3)

Incidence The association between sciatic neuropathy and hip arthroplasty is well established, with an incidence of approximately 1% to 2%.[7] The incidence of sciatic nerve injury in acetabular fracture repair is approximately 2.9%.[21] These diagnoses are clinical, and at least one study has shown that the prevalence of nerve changes seen with monitoring with transcranial motor and/ or somatosensory evoked potentials is greater than what is clinically identified.[2] In that study of 76 patients undergoing hip arthroscopy in the lateral position, 58% had intraoperative nerve dysfunction, whereas only 7% were diagnosed with a clinical nerve injury.

Predisposing factors The common peroneal component of the sciatic nerve is not only more commonly affected than the tibial portion but, when both portions are affected, the peroneal injury is also usually more severe.[1] Sudderland reported that, in 30% of the specimens that he has studied, the sciatic nerve exits the pelvis as 2 separate nerves. In such people, the tibial division will enter the gluteal region distal compared with the peroneal division. Also the peroneal component is the more lateral and superficial portion of the sciatic nerve; once separate, it is relatively more fixed between the sciatic notch and the fibular head. These anatomic reasons make the peroneal portion (or division) more vulnerable to injury, such as traction and compression from retractors.

Yet another proposed explanation is based on the morphologic differences between the tightly packed fascicles of the peroneal division and those of the tibial division, which have relatively more connective tissue.[3] The abundant connective tissue, as in the tibial division, protects those nerves and makes them less vulnerable to transection or compression than nerves with tightly packed fascicles such as in the peroneal division. Also, because the peroneal division nerve bundles are larger, in accord with Laplace's Law, they are at a higher risk of compression compared with tibial nerve bundles.

Another predisposing or risk factor to mention is patients who underwent hip fracture surgery, had preoperative traction before surgery, or had a longer duration of preoperative traction seem to have a higher risk of developing PPNTI.[8]

Mechanism of injury Common mechanisms of injury for hip procedures are either from the placement of posterior acetabular retractors or from anterior or lateral traction on the femur.[3,22] The posterior inferior acetabular retractor lies in close proximity to the sciatic nerve; during hip flexion, the nerve can impinge on the acetabular retractor. Traction of up to 40 to 57 kg may be necessary to sufficiently distract the joint for adequate visualization, and it can be very difficult to find the right balance between proper traction and not excessively stretching the nerve to the point of injury. Positions that cause hyperflexion, abduction, and extension of the leg results in stretching of nerves, which results in injury after a prolonged period of time. The evaluation of the function of the sciatic nerve through the intraoperative monitoring of somatosensory cortical evoked potentials has implicated limb positioning and retractor placement in nerve injuries.[6,23] In those cases, evoked potentials returned to baseline after the repositioning of retractors and/or limbs. Satcher and colleagues[22] used motor evoked potentials in combination with electromyography monitoring during revision THA in 27 consecutive patients and found changes in monitoring parameters associated with leg position, manipulation of acetabular allograft, and insertion of Kirschner (K) wires in the acetabulum, which returned to baseline after extending the hip or repositioning the acetabular allograft or K wires in all cases. In fact, in their study, leg positioning was the most commonly associated intraoperative factor causing changes in monitored parameters.

Another proposed mechanism in total hip replacement is excessive tension caused by lengthening of the extremity. In fact, in cases involving limb lengthening, there was a higher incidence of neuropathy, especially in limbs that were lengthened more than 2.5 cm.[1] However, when Nercessian looked at 1284 cases of THA of which 74% had some limb lengthening involved, he found only 1 case of iatrogenic nerve injury, which was caused by laceration and not traction.[13] There are, unfortunately, no guidelines regarding the amount of lengthening that can be achieved safely.

In the intraoperative monitoring study by Telleria and colleagues,[2] they concluded that maximum traction weight, not the total traction time, is the greatest risk factor for sciatic nerve dysfunction during hip arthroscopy. In their study, the odds of a nerve event increased 4% with every 0.45-kg increase in the traction amount. On the other hand, earlier studies have shown that total traction time was a significant risk factor for developing nerve traction injury, noting an absence of neurologic complications when traction time is limited to less than 2 hours.[24,25]

As mentioned, the peroneal portion of the sciatic is more commonly involved given its more lateral and superficial nature; in the lateral transtrochanteric approach, it would be difficult to compress the tibial portion without compressing the peroneal portion.[1] This point may account for the fact that when both divisions are injured, the peroneal injury is more severe.

In hip arthroscopy, the joint capsule often requires distraction forces to facilitate the introduction of the scope and instruments into the joint, necessary to visualize the innermost depths of the hip socket, but unfortunately also the mechanism of PPNTI if done for too long.[26]

Clinical presentation Injury manifests as paralysis of the hamstring muscles and all the muscles below the knee leading to weak knee flexion and foot drop. There is impairment of sensation below the knee with the exception of the medial aspect of the leg and foot.

Prevention and treatment Prevention of PPNTI of the sciatic nerve is not only dependent on good operative technique but also more on the need for constant attention to limb positioning,

placement of retractors, as well as the weight and duration of retraction. Keeping the amount of traction to less than 50 lb can help reduce the risk of nerve injury. Temporary repositioning of the limbs should be considered during lengthy operations. Traction should be kept to less than 2 hours, or the surgeon should attempt to identify situations when traction can be released or reduced to decrease tension on the nerve.[2,5,27] Tellerias's[2] intraoperative monitoring findings have shown that up to 75% of nerves have shown at least partial recovery after 15 minutes of rest. This rest may involve addressing the peripheral compartment first with minimal traction, removing negative pressure suction seal of the hip before initiating traction, increasing traction slowly with frequent fluoroscopic checks, or even performing capsulotomies. Some have recommended the use of tensiometers during surgery for careful monitoring of the distraction forces and the length of time they are applied.[28]

Given the risk of sciatic nerve injury during hip arthroplasty, some centers now routinely monitor for potential nerve injury with intraoperative monitoring using evoked potentials and free run electromyogram (EMG) to warn surgeons of potential peripheral nerve damage during surgery.[2,29] However, it remains controversial whether intraoperative nerve monitoring can prevent postoperative sequelae; at least one study found no difference in rates of nerve complications.[23]

In posterior acetabular retraction, the surgeon should try to keep the hip extended whenever possible. When there is extensive acetabular dissection and the use of structural allografts, the position of the sciatic nerve should be assessed carefully because these were associated with sciatic nerve compression.[22] Distraction forces may need to be modified in individual cases given the difference in the inherent laxity because too much force will likely result in hyperelongation of the leg and neuropraxia of the nerves at risk.[5]

Navarro and colleagues[11] came up with and recommended a 5-step surgical approach for reducing the incidence of sciatic nerve palsy: (1) direct finger palpation of the nerve within the posterior scar tissues; (2) limited sciatic neurolysis in difficult cases with extensive scarring; (3) retractor placement guided by the above; (4) final assessment by repeated palpation of the effects of the intraoperative changes in limb position on tension in the nerve and/or compression by a bony or prosthetic prominence; and (5) assessment of tension in the nerve or compression by a bony or prosthetic prominence during trial reduction and range-of-motion testing at the end of the case. In this study, they were able to decrease the incidence of sciatic nerve palsy by 50%. It should be mentioned that although limited sciatic neurolysis of nerves that are tethered or difficult to locate and increased intraoperative attention with palpation of the nerve before and after arthroplasty may help to decrease the prevalence of nerve injury, extra care must be taken because these techniques may also damage the anastomotic blood supply and cause increased scarring.

Others, such as Yacoubian and colleagues,[12] advocate routine visual sciatic nerve identification and tagging in revision hip surgery as one method to potentially reduce the risks of sciatic nerve injury, especially in hip revision given that scarred fibers of the gluteus maximus can easily be mistaken for the sciatic nerve, and relying solely on finger palpation may often be misleading. In the 350 cases in which this surgical technique was implemented, no permanent cases of sciatic nerve injury occurred.

Treatment has mostly been supportive and nonoperative. Physical therapy is prescribed to address motor deficits and prevent joint contractures. Orthoses are prescribed to treat foot drop, allowing clearance during the swing phase and preventing the steppage gait that indicates weak dorsiflexors and also help prevent equinus deformity. Select instances when surgical intervention may be considered include cases of documented limb lengthening, hematoma evacuation, or if there is suspicion of other mechanical causes of neuropathy.[15]

Pudendal nerve injury (S2–S4)

Incidence Amarenco and colleagues[30] calculated a total incidence of 2% of pudendal nerve injury secondary to an orthopedic operation. In hip arthroscopy, pudendal nerve injury may occur in as many as 10% of cases.[31] Locker and Beguin[32] reported the first 2 cases of pudendal neurapraxia in hip arthroscopy. Glick and colleagues[28] reported 4 pudendal nerve injuries in a series of 16 arthroscopies. Funke and Munzinger[9] reported 1 pudendal nerve injury in 19 cases. A meta-analysis by Byrd[10] found 10 neurapraxias in 1491 cases.

Predisposing factors This nerve is most vulnerable to injury at its distal anatomic course, where it runs upwards toward the pubic symphysis.[30]

Mechanism of injury Nerve compression is the most likely pathophysiological mechanism. When looking at pudendal neuropathy after femoral nailing, Brumback and colleagues[33] measured the pressure applied on the perineum and found a significant difference in the pressure/operative time ratio between groups with and without pudendal

neuropathy (73 kg/h vs 35 kg/h, respectively). They did not find a significant difference, however, in the operative time (168 minutes vs 158 minutes). The suggested mechanism of injury during hip arthroscopy might be compression of the rami during traction against the perineal post.

Clinical presentation Initially, there may be perineal and groin pain followed by a sensory deficit. In some cases, this deficit is associated with sexual disorders, such as impotence or anejaculation.

Prevention and treatment Recommendations for prevention or reducing the risk of pudendal nerve injury include limiting traction to only critical operative moment of operation and the use of good padding on the foot plate and in the perineum.[30] Lindenbaum and colleagues[34] showed that pressure on the perineum can be reduced by using a perineal post with a bigger diameter that provides better force distribution. The recommended diameter of the perineal post is 8 to 10 cm.[34,35] The ideal position of this perineal post is between the intact lower limb and the external genital organs.[34,36] Another recommended preventive measure is the ventral decubitus position on the fracture table.[34,35]

Femoral nerve injury (L2–4)

Incidence The femoral nerve is rarely injured after primary hip arthroplasty, (0.04%–2.6% of cases)[37,38] and in general have been more common in obstetric and pelvic surgeries (most caused by self-retaining retractors[38]) than in orthopedic procedures.[37] Although considered rare, it is likely underreported because it is frequently self-limiting.[39] The incidence is higher in revision surgery ranging in 1.0% to 7.6% of cases.[37,38]

Predisposing factors After passing beneath the inguinal ligament, the femoral nerve is in close proximity to the femoral head and acetabular rim, the tendon insertion of the vastus intermedius, the psoas tendon, the hip, and the joint capsule. At this level, there is little protection to the femoral nerve from retractors.[37,40] This fact may explain why there is higher incidence of femoral neuropathy in lateral and anterolateral approaches to the hip joint.[37,41] The left femoral nerve may be more vulnerable to ischemic injury because of the greater number of branches and richer anastomosis of the deep circumflex iliac artery on the right.[38]

The fascicular architecture of the femoral nerve may also contribute to its low susceptibility to injury because as the anterior division fibers travel separately in a flat fascicle situated ventromedially within the nerve, they may be more exposed to trauma within the pelvis; at the same time, they are less likely to sustain PPNTI caused by orthopedic surgery.[42]

Mechanism of injury Procedures that require the lower extremity to be positioned in an acutely flexed, abducted, and externally rotated position for long periods can cause traction injury and also compression by angling the femoral nerve beneath the inguinal ligament. Prolonged retraction exposure of the hip, in an anterior or anterolateral approach, is also a mechanism of retractor-induced injury.[37,41] Improper placement of the anterior acetabular retractor as the tip of the Hohmann retractor is placed near the femoral nerve is a commonly cited mechanism of femoral nerve injury.[43,44] Simmons and colleagues[40] concluded that all femoral neuropathies in their series were secondary to retractor placement with direct compression of the nerve. In THA, the femoral nerve is most at risk during placement of anterior acetabular retractors when anterior or anterolateral approaches are used.[3] Limb lengthening may endanger the nerve through stretch, although the sciatic rather than the femoral nerve is particularly at risk with this procedure.[45]

Clinical presentation The classic presentation is diminished or lost sensation in the distribution of the saphenous nerve (anterior thigh and medial aspect of the leg) with weak hip flexion and loss of extension of the knee. Decreased or absent patellar reflex may also be present.

Prevention and treatment There should be care taken with positioning patients and limb maneuvering. Exaggerated hip flexion, abduction, and external rotation should be avoided. Temporary repositioning of the limbs should be considered during lengthy operations. In an anterolateral approach, placing the tip of the retractor against the acetabular margin needs to be avoided.[46]

Treatment is partly dictated by the suspected mechanism and severity of injury, and prompt and accurate diagnosis is very important. A compressive hematoma may need drainage and any underlying coagulopathy corrected. Surgical exploration is indicated for injuries that fail to show adequate signs of recovery within about 3 months.[37] This exploration may include repair, grafting, or neurolysis. Nonoperative management should include physical therapy to prevent muscle atrophy and reduce the risk of deep vein thrombosis. A removable brace, such as a knee immobilizer, to hold the knee in extension should be used to prevent contracture and allow safe ambulation.

Following Knee Surgery

Peroneal nerve injury (L4–5 S1–2)

Incidence Peroneal nerve injury causing foot drop is a well-known complication of total knee arthroplasty. The incidence varies from 0% to 9.5%.[47] The overall incidence of perioperative injury is estimated to be 0.79%.[48] Again, more than one etiologic factor including PPNTI exist for peroneal nerve injury, and the cause is unknown in most cases.[49] True incidence may be in the higher range because of the presence of atypical peroneal nerve impairments that have different symptoms.[50]

Predisposing factors The common peroneal nerve is most susceptible when it courses around the fibular neck and passes through the fibroosseous opening in the superficial head of the peroneus longus muscle. This opening can be quite tough and can result in the nerve angulating through it at an acute angle. Also, significant fibrous connective tissue secures the nerve to this proximal portion of the fibula, potentially compromising the nerve. The common peroneal nerve may also be more susceptible to traction injuries because it is relatively more fixed between the sciatic notch and the fibular head.

A valgus deformity of the knee joint of at least 10° is a known risk factor for peroneal PPNTI.[51–53] A preoperative flexion contracture of the knee is another predisposing factor because it increases stretch on the nerve.[53] However, not all studies found that flexion contractures or valgus deformities were significant risk factors for the development of peroneal nerve palsy.[47,54] Postoperative epidural analgesia may be another significant risk factor for the development of PPNTI of the peroneal nerve.[51,53,55] The thought is that epidural analgesia may cause patients to inadvertently rest the limb in a position that directly compresses the peroneal nerve at the fibular head.[48] As mentioned earlier, rheumatoid arthritis is another known risk factor for peroneal nerve PPNTI, although some question if the risk is directly from the effect of rheumatoid arthritis or caused by sequelae of the disease that are themselves risk factors (eg, preoperative valgus deformity and flexion contracture).[56] The length of tourniquet use may be another risk factor, with a total tourniquet time greater than 120 minutes thought to be a significant risk factor for neuropathy.[51]

Mechanism of injury Intraoperative correction of a valgus deformity of the knee results in traction on the peroneal nerve and PPNTI.[48,52] The stretch of the nerve and the surrounding soft tissues that occurs during correction of valgus deformity and flexion contracture is thought to result in compromised blood supply to the nerve and subsequent injury.[48] Lateral position is a common risk factor because the nerve is potentially compressed at the fibular head. The nerve is also at risk from compression over the fibular head by an external agent, such as the continuous passive motion machine.[47] The mechanism of injury caused by tourniquet use seems to be caused by both ischemia and mechanical deformation.[48] EMG changes were seen in up to 75% of patients in studies of patients whose surgery was performed with the use of pneumatic tourniquet.[48] What is still uncertain is whether the EMG changes were clinically significant. Other studies have not shown a significant relationship between tourniquet pressure/duration and nerve injury.[47,53] Nevertheless, the common recommendation is to limit tourniquet use to 2 hours or less because most studies performed to identify the risk factor for peroneal nerve injury after total knee arthroplasty did not find the use of a tourniquet to be a significant factor if the duration was 2 hours or less.[51]

Clinical presentation Commonly, patients with motor deficits, such as weakness or even absence of ankle dorsiflexion or extension of the great toe, will result in foot drop or dragging of the toes during ambulation. Sensory manifestations are described along the anterolateral border of the leg and the dorsum of the digits except those supplied by saphenous and sural nerves.

It is important to note that some patients may not present with the typical peroneal nerve palsy symptoms yet still have a peroneal nerve injury. These patients present with mild atypical symptoms, and their only clinical manifestation of peroneal nerve injury may include difficulty with rehabilitation, achieving suboptimal range of motion, or persistent transient symptoms that interfere with their daily activities.[50]

Prevention and treatment If a PPNTI is suspected, the knee should be repositioned to 20° to 30° of flexion and any constrictive dressing should be changed to relieve traction or possible local compression.[47,48] This practice is followed with physical therapy and nonsteroidal antiinflammatory drugs/neuroleptics for any pain. Surgical exploration is recommended for any patient not showing either clinical resolution or EMG improvement after 3 months, especially in patients with more severe injuries.[57]

DIAGNOSIS OF PPTNI

A thorough history and clinical examination are essential to localize the lesion and to identify a preexisting peripheral neuropathy. The clinical examination serves to identify whether single or multiple nerves are involved and the impairment severity of motor, sensory, or both, which is of prognostic value. Pain is common after surgery; because of that, pain can often mask nerve injury–associated pain as well as the associated loss of movement and sensation. One retrospective study of 612 cases of iatrogenic injury to peripheral nerves acknowledges that too many patients were inappropriately sent to pain clinics, and ineffective treatment led to delay in appropriate diagnosis and treatment.[58] This finding is unfortunate because in those cases that might need repair, delay is associated with a poor outcome after the repair.[59] In the same study, delay in recognition and, therefore, treatment was a cause of litigation and contributed to the poor outcome in many cases. If a deficit is found, electrophysiological and imaging studies are performed and early consultation with a physiatrist or neurologist is advisable.

EMG and Nerve Conduction Studies

EMG involves insertion of a needle electrode into a muscle that is being tested and recording the electrical activity of that muscle both at rest and during voluntary activation. In PPNTI, there are reduced numbers of functioning axons, which results in a reduction in the number of motor units recruited. Abnormal spontaneous activity (eg, fibrillation potentials, positive sharp waves) takes 1 to 4 weeks to develop and disappears with reinnervation. If they are present early on, it may imply a preexisting condition, and a specific diagnosis of the cause would not be able to be made.

Nerve conduction studies (NCSs) are used to assess the function of motor and sensory nerves by measuring nerve conduction velocity and the size of the muscle response. These values help estimate the number of axons and muscle fibers that get activated with each stimulus. NCSs evaluate the functional integrity of peripheral nerves and enable localization of focal lesions. NCSs can differentiate between an axonal loss versus demyelinating pathologic process and can also be helpful in ruling out a subclinical neuropathy. NCSs and EMG are complementary and can help to determine the basis of the clinical deficit; localize the lesion; determine whether a lesion is complete or incomplete; define the severity and age of the lesion; and guide prognosis and course of recovery.

In the setting of clinical weakness, electrodiagnostics can be very helpful in guiding patient education and care. A more poor outcome is expected if there are electrophysiologic signs of axonotmesis or neurotmesis: extensive fibrillation potentials and positive sharp waves with no or few motor unit action potentials recruited with maximal effort. A more favorable outcome is expected if there are electrophysiologic signs of neuropraxia: no fibrillations or positive sharp waves noted in the presence of conduction block on NCSs.

Timing of electrodiagnostic testing is critical. Abnormal spontaneous activity is noted in nearby muscles if there is axon loss as soon as 1 week after injury; muscles further away from site of injury may not show abnormality until 3 weeks after injury.

Imaging Studies

The current recommendation is to do a 3-T magnetic resonance imaging that provides adequate resolution to visualize peripheral nerves and also help identify and confirm the site of the lesion. High-resolution ultrasound has also been proposed as an adjunct to electrodiagnosis.[60]

PREVENTION AND TREATMENT

A peripheral nerve injury is one of the most distressing complications of surgery. There is no amount of time spent in consultative discussion concerning surgical complications that will decrease the high degree of dissatisfaction that is expressed by these patients. By all other measures, the surgery may have been a success, but patients' dissatisfaction will often preclude a good rating of the result. Because PPNTI is likely the most preventable perioperative complication, it is essential that everything is done to reduce it. A sound knowledge of anatomy and the risks posed by positioning patients and their limbs for surgery and retraction is essential in understanding PPNTI prevention. A careful surgeon has to be familiar with the anatomy of the nerves in the vicinity of a planned procedure. There has to be allowance for any variations encountered in the course of the operation. Nerves that are particularly at risk may need to be exposed, and this may require that a longer incision is made. A thorough preoperative history is important to identify conditions that predispose patients to nerve injury, such as diabetes, hypertension, smoking, and rheumatoid arthritis. Time should be taken to do a good physical examination to assess for any preexisting neurologic dysfunction. Attention should be given to avoid intraoperative hypotension, hypothermia, and dehydration. Other than careful positioning of patients, important perioperative care to reduce the risk of PPNTI includes protective padding, padded arm boards, and

avoidance of contact with hard surfaces or any direct pressure to susceptible peripheral nerves. Traction weight should be kept at less than 50 lb and for no longer than 2 hours[4,5,61] or released intermittently for prolonged cases. Perioperative continuous nerve monitoring may also be an important preventative measure for difficult cases. A simple postoperative assessment of extremity nerve function is crucial because it may lead to early recognition of peripheral nerve injury and better prognosis. To involve patients early on and allow them to be an ally in maximizing recovery cannot be emphasized enough. It is, therefore, highly recommended that as soon as an PPNTI is diagnosed, patients are not only informed but also involved in a thorough discussion regarding the nerve injury and prognosis.

REFERENCES

1. Schmalzried TP, Amstutz HC, Dorey FJ. Nerve palsy associated with total hip replacement. J Bone Joint Surg Am 1991;73A:1074–80.
2. Telleria JJ, Safran MR, Gardi JN, et al. Risk of sciatic nerve traction injury during hip arthroscopy-Is it the amount or duration? J Bone Joint Surg Am 2012;22:2025–32.
3. DeHart MM, Riley LH. Nerve Injuries in total hip arthroplasty. J Am Acad Orthop Surg 1999;7:101–11.
4. Clarke MT, Villar RN. Hip arthroscopy: complications in 1054 cases. Clin Orthop Relat Res 2003;406:84–8.
5. Sampson TG. Complications of hip arthroscopy. Tech Orthop 2005;20:63–6.
6. Nercessian OA, Gonzalez EG, Stinchfield FE. The use of somatosensory evoked potential during revision or reoperation for total hip arthroplasty. Clin Orthop 1989;243:138–42.
7. Schmalzried TP, Noordin S, Amstutz HC. Update on nerve palsy associated with total hip replacement. Clin Orthop Relat Res 1997;344:188–206.
8. Kemler MA, de Vries M, van der Tol A. Duration of preoperative traction associated with sciatic neuropathy after hip fracture surgery. Clin Orthop Relat Res 2006;556:230–2.
9. Funke EL, Munzinger U. Complications in hip arthroscopy. Arthroscopy 1996;12:156–9.
10. Byrd JW. Complications associated with hip arthroscopy. In: Byrd JW, editor. Operative arthroscopy. New York: Thieme; 1998. p. 171–6.
11. Navarro RA, Schmalzired TP, Amstutz HC, et al. Surgical approach and nerve palsy in total hip arthroplasty. J Arthroplasty 1995;10:1.
12. Yacoubian SV, Sah AP, Estok DM. Incidence of sciatic nerve palsy after revision hip arthroplasty through a posterior approach. J Arthroplasty 2010;25(1):31–4.

13. Nercessian OA, Piccoluga F, Eftekhar NS. Posoperative sciatic and femoral nerve palsy with reference to leg lengthening and medicalization/lateralization of the hip joint following total hip arthroplasty. Clin Orthop Relat Res 1994;304:165–71.

14. Johanson NA, Pellicci PM, Tsairis P, et al. Nerve injury in total hip arthroplasty. Clin Orthop 1983; 179:214–22.

15. Brown GD, Swanson EA, Nercessian OA. Neurologic injuries after total hip arthroplasty. Am J Orthop 2008;37(4):191–7.

16. Farrell CM, Springer BD, Haidukewych GJ, et al. Motor nerve palsy following primary total hip arthroplasty. J Bone Joint Surg Am 2005;87A(12):2619–25.

17. Nercessian OA, Macaulay W, Stinchfield FE. Peripheral neuropathies following total hip arthroplasty. J Arthroplasty 1994;9:645–51.

18. Solheim LF, Hagen R. Femoral and sciatic neuropathies after total hip arthroplasty. Acta Orthop Scand 1980;51(3):531–4.

19. Edwards BN, Tullos HS, Noble PC. Contributory factors and etiology of sciatic nerve palsy in total hip arthroplasty. Clin Orthop 1987;218:136–41.

20. Al-Ajmi A, Rouseff RT, Khuraibet A. Iatrogenic femoral neuropathy: two cases and literature update. J Clin Neuromuscul Dis 2010;12(2):66–75.

21. Haidukewych GJ, Scaduto J, Herscovici D, et al. Iatrogenic nerve injury in acetabular fracture surgery: a comparison of monitored and unmonitored procedures. J Orthop Trauma 2002;16(5):297–301.

22. Satcher RL, Noss RS, Yingling CD, et al. The use of motor-evoked potentials to monitor sciatic nerve status during revision total hip arthroplasty. J Arthroplasty 2003;18(3):329–32.

23. Black DL, Reckling FW, Porter SS. Somatosensory evoked potential monitored during total hip arthroplasty. Clin Orthop 1991;262:170–7.

24. O'Leary JA, Berend K, Vail TP. The relationship between diagnosis and outcome in arthroscopy of the hip. Arthroscopy 2001;17(2):181–8.

25. Philippon M, Schenker M, Briggs K, et al. Femoroacetabular impingement in 45 professional athletes: associated pathologies and return to sport following arthroscopic decompression. Knee Surg Sports Traumatol Arthrosc 2007;15(7):908–14.

26. Dorfmann H, Boyer T. Arthroscopy of the hip: 12 years of experience. Arthroscopy 1999;15(1):67–72.

27. Lo YP, Chan YS, Lien LC, et al. Complications of hip arthroscopy: analysis of seventy three cases. Chang Gung Med J 2006;29(1):86–92.

28. Glick JM, Sampson TG, Gordon RB, et al. Hip arthroscopy by the lateral approach. Arthroscopy 1987;3:4–12.

29. Saidha S, Spillane J, Mullins G, et al. Spectrum of peripheral neuropathies associated with surgical interventions; A neurophysiological assessment. J Brachial Plex Peripher Nerve Inj 2010;5:1–4.

30. Amarenco G, Ismael SS, Bayle B, et al. Electrophyiological analysis of pudendal neuropathy following traction. Muscle Nerve 2001;24:116–9.

31. Merrell G, Medvecky M, Daigneault J, et al. Hip arthroscopy without a perineal post: a safer technique for hip distraction. Arthroscopy 2007;23(1): 107e1–3.

32. Locker B, Beguin J. L'arthrscopie de hanche. J Med Lyon 1984;1304:25–6.

33. Brumback RJ, Ellison TS, Molligan H, et al. Pudendal nerve palsy complicating intramedullary nailing of the femur. J Bone Joint Surg Am 1992; 74:1450–5.

34. Lindenbaum SD, Fleming LL, Smith DW. Pudendal nerve palsies associated with closed intramedullary femoral fixation. A report of two cases and a study of the mechanism of injury. J Bone Joint Surg Am 1982;64:934–8.

35. Kao JT, Burton D, Comstock C, et al. Pudendal nerve palsy after intramedullary nailing. J Orthop Trauma 1993;7:58–63.

36. France MP, Aurori BF. Pudendal nerve palsy following fracture table traction. Clin Orthop 1992; 276:272–6.

37. Moore AE, Stringer MD. Iatrogenic femoral nerve injury: a systematic review. Surg Radiol Anat 2011;33:649–58.

38. Boontje AH, Haaxma R. Femoral neuropathy as a complication of aortic surgery. J Cardiovasc Surg 1987;28:286–9.

39. Brasch RC, Bufo AJ, Kreienberg PF, et al. Femoral neuropathy secondary to the use of a self-retaining retractor. Report of three cases and review of the literature. Dis Colon Rectum 1995;38:1115–8.

40. Simmons C Jr, Izant TH, Rothman RH, et al. Femoral neuropathy following total hip arthroplasty. Anatomic study, case reports, and literature review. J Arthroplasty 1991;(Suppl 6):S57–66.

41. Van der Linde MJ, Tonino AJ. Nerve injury after hip arthroplasty. 5/600 cases after uncemented hip replacement, anterolateral approach versus direct lateral approach. Acta Orthop Scand 1997;68:521–3.

42. Gustafson KJ, Pinault GC, Neville JJ, et al. Fascicular anatomy of human femoral nerve: implications for neural prostheses using nerve cuff electrodes. J Rehabil Res Dev 2009;46:973–84.

43. Wasielewski RC, Crossett LS, Rubash HE. Neural and vascular injury in total hip arthroplasty. Orthop Clin North Am 1992;23(2):219–35.

44. Heller KD, Prescher A, Birnbaum K, et al. Femoral nerve lesion in total hip replacement: an experimental study. Arch Orthop Trauma Surg 1998; 117(3):153–5.

45. Eggli S, Hankemayer S, Müller ME. Nerve palsy after leg lengthening in total replacement arthroplasty for developmental dysplasia of the hip. J Bone Joint Surg Br 1999;81:843–5.

46. Slater N, Singh R, Senasinghe N, et al. Pressure monitoring of the femoral nerve during total hip replacement: an explanation for iatropathic palsy. J R Coll Surg Edinb 2000;45:231–3.

47. Schinsky MF, Macaulay W, Parks ML, et al. Nerve injury after primary total knee arthroplasty. J Arthroplasty 2001;16:1048–54.

48. Nercessian OA, Ugwonali OF, Park S. Peroneal nerve palsy after total knee arthroplasty. J Arthroplasty 2005;20:1068–73.

49. Asp JP, Rand JA. Peroneal nerve palsy after total knee arthroplasty. Clin Orthop Relat Res 1990; 261:233.

50. Zywiel MG, Mont MA, McGrath MS, et al. Peroneal nerve dysfunction after total knee arthroplasty. J Arthroplasty 2011;26(3):379–85.

51. Horlocker TT, Cabanela ME, Wedel DJ. Does postoperative epidural analgesia increase the risk of peroneal nerve palsy after total knee arthroplasty? Anesth Analg 1994;79:495.

52. Kinghorn K, Ellinas H, Barboi AC, et al. Case scenario: nerve injury after knee arthroplasty and sciatic nerve block. Anesthesiology 2012;116(4):918–23.

53. Idusuyi OB, Morrey BF. Peroneal nerve palsy after total knee arthroplasty. Assessment of predisposing and prognostic factors. J Bone Joint Surg Am 1996; 78:177–84.

54. Miyasaka KC, Ranawat CS, Mullaji A. 10- to 20-year follow-up of total knee arthroplasty for valgus deformities. Clin Orthop 1997;345:29.

55. Cohen EE, Van Duker B, Siegel S, et al. Common peroneal nerve palsy associated with epidural analgesia. Anesth Analg 1993;76:429.

56. Knutson K, Leden I, Sturfelt G, et al. Nerve palsy after knee arthroplasty in patients with rheumatoid arthritis. Scand J Rheumatol 1983; 12(3):201.

57. Krackow KA, Maar DC, Mont MA, et al. Surgical decompression for peroneal nerve palsy after total knee arthroplasty. Clin Orthop 1993;292:223.

58. Khan R, Birch R. Iatropathic injuries of peripheral nerves. J Bone Joint Surg Br 2001;83:1145–8.

59. Birch R, Raji AR. Repair of median and ulnar nerves: primary suture is best. J Bone Joint Surg Br 1991;73-B:154–7.

60. Lakhen AG. Perioperative peripheral nerve injuries. Cont Educ Anaesth Crit Care Pain 2011;1–5.

61. Ilizaliturri VM Jr, Chaidez PA, Aguilera JM, et al. Special instruments and techniques for hip arthroscopy. Tech Orthop 2005;20:9–16.

Spondylopelvic Dissociation

Matthew P. Sullivan, MD[a], Harvey E. Smith, MD[b],
James M. Schuster, MD, PhD[c], Derek Donegan, MD[a],
Samir Mehta, MD[a,d], Jaimo Ahn, MD, PhD[a,*]

KEYWORDS

- Spondylopelvic dissociation • Transverse sacral fracture • Lumbosacral dissociation
- Spinopelvic dissociation • U-type sacral fracture • Atypical sacral fracture • Polytrauma
- Triangular osteosynthesis

KEY POINTS

- Spondylopelvic dissociation is a rare and highly complex injury pattern resulting in multiplanar instability of the lumbopelvis. Hallmarks include bilateral vertical sacral fractures with a horizontal component. Iliolumbosacral instability occurs in both the coronal and the axial planes.
- Extreme axial load is required to produce this injury pattern resulting in bony deformity as well as soft tissue trauma. Common mechanisms of injury include suicide jumps, motor vehicle and motorcycle collisions, and under-vehicle explosions.
- Diagnosis relies on thin-section computed tomographic scan with coronal and sagittal reconstructions.
- Surgical treatment has evolved greatly over the past 15 to 20 years and both percutaneous and open options are available. Triangular osteosynthesis is the most relied on method of fixation as it controls deformity in both sagittal and axial planes.
- The role of fracture reduction and nerve root decompression is debated in literature.

SPECTRUM OF DISEASE: HISTORICAL PERSPECTIVE

Spondylopelvic dissociation is a complex injury pattern that has recently increased in prevalence as the United States Armed Forces have engaged in conflict in Iraq and Afghanistan.[1,2] These high-energy injuries are the least understood of the sacral fractures and inconsistencies in nomenclature have contributed to the confusion within the literature. They are most frequently seen in suicide jumpers, blast injuries, and high-speed motor vehicle collisions. Spondylopelvic dissociation is at the extreme end of the spectrum of atypical sacral fractures (eg, transverse and U-type sacral

fractures) and is a relatively new term. It was preceded by the term transverse sacral fracture and the first case report of a transverse sacral fracture was published in 1969.[3] Since that time, their representation in the literature has been somewhat limited.[4–13] Roy-Camille and colleagues[7] published their landmark paper describing in detail the anatomy, pathoanatomy, and biomechanics of transverse sacral fractures in 1985. In addition, they proposed the first classification scheme for this fracture pattern.

As advanced imaging modalities and surgeons' understanding of transverse sacral fractures improved, the term U-shaped sacral fracture emerged. This fracture pattern was introduced in

[a] Department of Orthopaedic Surgery, Hospital of the University of Pennsylvania, University of Pennsylvania, 3400 Spruce Street, Philadelphia, PA 19143, USA; [b] Department of Orthopaedic Surgery, Pennsylvania Hospital, University of Pennsylvania, 800 Spruce Street, Philadelphia, PA 19107, USA; [c] Department of Neurological Surgery, Hospital of the University of Pennsylvania, 3400 Spruce Street, Philadelphia, PA 19143, USA; [d] Division of Orthopaedic Trauma, Department of Orthopaedic Surgery, Hospital of the University of Pennsylvania, University of Pennsylvania, 3400 Spruce Street, Philadelphia, PA 19143, USA
* Corresponding author.
E-mail address: Jaimo.Ahn@uphs.upenn.edu

Orthop Clin N Am 45 (2014) 65–75
http://dx.doi.org/10.1016/j.ocl.2013.08.002

1996 by Ebraheim and colleagues[14] in which they described the injury as a "transverse fracture at the S2-S3 segment and the longitudinal fractures running on either side through the sacral foramina." Since that time, there have been few published reports in the English language describing the U-shaped sacral fracture pattern, with all publications being either case reports, case series, or expert opinion.[15–23] In addition to U-shaped sacral fractures, H-shaped, T-shaped, and Y-shaped sacral fractures have been described, all of which include both transverse and vertical components.[2,13,19,24]

Around the time U-shaped sacral fractures surfaced in the literature, spondylopelvic dissociation made its appearance as a distinct and highly complex type of U-shaped sacral fracture in which considerable displacement exists between the cephalad superior-central sacrum segment/lumbar spine and the caudal bilateral sacral alae and inferior sacral segments.[25] In similar fashion to U-shaped sacral fractures there is scant literature beyond case series and literature reviews describing this injury pattern.[1,2,19,26–30]

A close examination of the literature suggests the above-mentioned entities are in fact a spectrum of injury patterns with considerable overlap. Furthermore, there is spectrum of variability with respect to the nomenclature of these injuries. Reports describing similar injury patterns use multiple terms including transverse sacral fractures,[7] U-shaped sacral fractures,[15] spondylopelvic dissociation,[25] spinopelvic dissociation,[27] lumbopelvic dissociation,[29] and lumbosacral dissociation.[1]

CLASSIFICATION

Classically, sacral fractures have been classified by either the Roy-Camille system[7] or the Denis system,[9] although modifications exist.[8,13,31] Roy-Camille and colleagues[7] presented the first classification system for transverse sacral fractures in 1985. In this scheme there are 3 subtypes of injuries based on the mechanism and orientation of displacement (**Fig. 1**). Type 1 injury is a flexion deformity of the upper sacral segments onto the lower sacral segments without displacement. Type 2 injury is a flexion injury with posterior displacement of the superior segments relative to the inferior segments. Type 3 injury is an extension type injury with anterior displacement of the superior segments relative to the inferior segments. The Roy-Camille system fails to consider the level at which the transverse fracture takes place and this has important implications with respect to lumbopelvic stability, neurologic injury, and treatment algorithms.

The well-known Denis Classification of sacral fractures does not specifically address transverse sacral fractures; however, it incorporates these injuries into the zone 3 pattern, involving the central sacral canal.[9] Similarly, this system fails to describe the complex pathoanatomy seen in the spectrum of spondylopelvic dissociation effectively.

Only recently was the complex spectrum of spondylopelvic dissociation addressed in a comprehensive classification system that incorporates multiple facets of this disease.[1] Lehman and colleagues[1] proposed the Lumbosacral Injury Classification

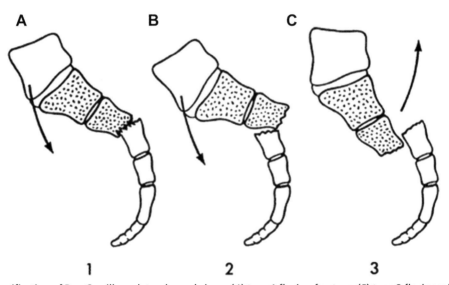

Fig. 1. Classification of Roy-Camille on lateral sacral views: (*A*) type 1 flexion fracture, (*B*) type 2 flexion with posterior displacement, and (*C*) type 3 extension with anterior displacement. (*From* Hunt N, Jennings A, Smith M. Current management of U-shaped sacral fractures or spino-pelvic dissociation. Injury 2002;33(2):123–6; with permission.)

System (LSICS) to address the deficiencies of the classification systems described above. Their work followed the large increase they observed in soldiers sustaining spondylopelvic dissociation injuries related to conflicts in the Middle East. The LSICS is based on a composite injury severity score that takes into account injury morphology, integrity of the posterior ligament complex, neurologic status, and the following 3 clinical modifiers: systemic injury load, soft tissue status, and expected mobility status. LSICS should be used to make management decisions for transverse sacral fracture with associated bilateral longitudinal components (U-/H-/T-/Y-shaped sacral fractures), traumatic spondylolisthesis at L5/S1, and vertically unstable sacral fracture. This system does not consider bilateral sacroiliac joint dislocations, because these injuries classically are considered pelvic ring injuries. A composite injury severity score is determined based on the injury morphology, integrity of the posterior ligament complex, and neurologic status. Operative treatment is then recommended based on this score in conjunction with the presence or absence of clinical modifiers (**Fig. 2**).

ANATOMY AND BIOMECHANICS

The sacrum forms from the fusion of 5 vertebral bodies and intervertebral disks. Completion of fusion takes place between ages 25 and 33 years of age. In the nontraumatized patient the lumbosacropelvic articulations are inherently stable due to bony engineering and ligamentous restraints. The V-shaped sacrum is wedged between the iliac bones bilaterally in both the axial and the coronal planes. The broad sacroiliac articulation superiorly gives way to narrowing distally. This articulation includes sacral segments 1 and 2.[13] Anteroinferiorly there is a shelf of dense cortical ilium blocking translation of the sacrum onto the pelvis.[4]

Furthermore, the dense posterior ligamentous structures provide support in addition to the bony restraints described. These structures are critical to the prevention of anterior translation and flexion of the sacrum as well as radially directed instability throughout the pelvis. The ligamentous structures are many in number. Pelvic ring stability is provided by the posterior, interosseous (and to a lesser extent anterior) sacroiliac ligaments, sacrospinous ligaments, and sacrotuberous ligaments. Lumbosacral stability is imparted by the supraspinous ligament, ligamentum flavum, interspinous ligament, iliolumbar ligament, lateral lumbosacral ligament, and the L5/S1 facet joint capsule. In concert, these dense soft tissue restraints behave like a posterior tension band, stabilizing the iliolumbosacral junctions from progressive deformity. Assessment and

understanding of the integrity of these structures are critical to managing spondylopelvic dissociation properly.[1]

Sacral neural foraminal anatomy has important clinical implications as well. S1 and S2 nerve roots occupy between one-quarter and one-third of the entire cross-sectional area of the respective foramina. Meanwhile, the lower nerve roots occupy roughly one-sixth of cross-sectional area of their foramina, which has important implications when considering nerve root decompression and removal of bony fracture debris.[13]

König and colleagues[21] describe the 2 over-riding biomechanical components of spondylopelvic dissociation. The first is the high-energy axial load resulting in the bilateral vertical components. This vertical instability causes the central component to pivot in flexion or extension, resulting in the transverse fracture line, usually occurring between S1 and S2 and causing the upper sacral segments to remain attached to the spine and the lower sacral segment to remain attached to the pelvis.

Critically important to fracture anatomy is the mechanism of injury and the forces imparted through the sacrum at the time of impact. Transverse sacral fractures can be thought of as flexion type (types 1 and 2) or extension type (type 3). As previously mentioned, Roy-Camille and colleagues[7] initially proposed this classification in 1985. They correlated their cadaveric biomechanical findings with clinical findings. From this they proposed that an axial load on the body with the lumbar spine in kyphosis results in flexion deformity. The superior sacral segment may translate posteriorly if enough energy is imparted through the system.[1] Conversely, with the lumbar spine in lordosis, the sacrum extends and the superior segment translates anteriorly. Pure axial compression of the sacrum occurs when the lumbar spine maintains its neutral alignment during impact. The blast or shear pattern has only recently been described. Blast morphology is characterized by extensive comminution of the proximal sacral segments. The typical mechanism for this injury is an under-vehicle explosion resulting in a superiorly directed force to the dorsal aspect of the sacrum. There is often massive soft tissue injury and they are frequently open injuries.[1,2,29,31]

CLINICAL EVALUATION AND RELATED CONSIDERATIONS

Because of the rarity of spondylopelvic dissociation, the initial diagnosis can be easily missed. For instance, transverse sacral fractures account for less than 5% of all sacral fractures.[5,13,15]

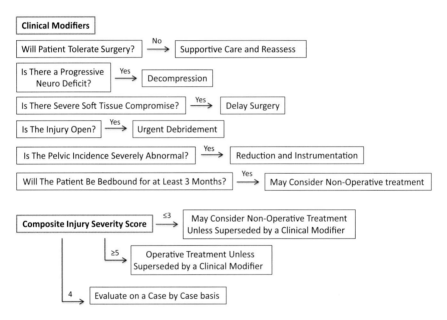

Fig. 2. The Lumbosarcal Injury Classification System (LSICS) offers a comprehensive approach for treatment strategies in spondylopelvic dissociation injuries. It includes a composite injury severity score and additional clinical modifiers.

Furthermore, greater than 95% of patients with this injury are polytraumatized with various other visceral and musculoskeletal injuries.[2,20,21,26] Additional pelvic ring injuries and spine injuries are common and seen in 44.4% and 31.7% of patients, respectively.[21] The communicative patient may describe sacrococcygeal pain and discomfort. As always, a detailed trauma evaluation following the Advance Trauma Life Support guidelines is essential. A detailed examination of the pelvic soft tissue envelope and musculoskeletal system should be performed, paying particular attention to the posterior soft tissue.[1,21] Morel-Lavallee (internal degloving) injury is common and may be suggested by a subcutaneous fluid collection or large ecchymotic patch over the sacrum.[21] Not only is this injury important to consider because it is known to greatly increase infection risk with and without surgery, but operative approaches and orthopedic instrumentation should avoid crossing these lesions. Palpation of the sacrum for a step-off and crepitation should be carefully performed. As with all high-energy lumbopelvic injuries, an anogenital examination must be performed to assess for occult open fractures. Open fracture through rectal or vaginal tissue mandates urgent debridement.

As expected, there is an exceedingly high rate of neurologic injury seen in spondylopelvic dissociation. Motor and sensory radicular deficits should be expected. In their seminal work, Roy-Camille and colleagues[7] reported some element of neurologic deficit in 100% of patients in their series. Similarly, high numbers have been reported in more recent reports of U-shaped sacral fractures.[20] In their systematic review, König and colleagues[21] describe greater than 94% of patients having some form of abnormal neurologic examination—44% of which developed bowel and/or bladder dysfunction—and included sexual dysfunction and dysesthesias.[1] The significance of this finding cannot be overstated, mandating the vigilant practice of thorough rectal and perirectal examination on presentation to the trauma bay. In addition, neural involvement may present as a mononeuropathy, oligoneuropathy, or cauda equina syndrome.

The ubiquitous neurologic injuries described may only be applicable to transverse component fractures that involve the upper sacral segments.[10,32] Sabiston and Wing[10] reported on 11 patients who sustained low sacral transverse fractures. Only 1 patient developed a neurologic deficit, whereas 5 of 5 patients with upper segment fractures developed deficits. To further complicate the clinical picture, significant nerve root injury may be present with normal lower extremity motor findings. The lower sacral nerve roots cannot be simply evaluated by testing lower extremity strength. A cursory skeletal trauma examination may miss neurologic injury below S1. As such, once stabilized, the patient should receive a thorough tertiary neurologic examination.

Complete neurologic recovery occurs in only 46.5% of patients with abnormal immediate post-injury neurologic examination, whereas failure to recover any lost function may be seen in upward of 21.9%.[21] The need and utility of surgical nerve root decompression in the acute setting continue to be debated in the literature.

RADIOGRAPHIC ASSESSMENT

The standard radiographic evaluation of spondylopelvic dissociation is notoriously difficult, which has accounted for the high rate of missed injuries before current advanced imaging techniques that are now becoming commonplace in all modern trauma centers. Nearly all of the early publications reporting on transverse sacral fractures describe these diagnostic difficulties as they relate to standard film interpretation.[3–5,7,8] That being said, there are subtle clues that the attuned observer can pick up to aid in the diagnosis. As part of the trauma series of radiographs, the anteroposterior view of the pelvis should be examined closely for 4 characteristic yet subtle findings, including L5 transverse process fractures, bilateral transforaminal or vertical alar sacral fractures, irregularities in the sacral foraminal lines, and paradoxic inlet view of the upper sacral bodies (**Fig. 3**). A lateral view of the sacrum can confirm the diagnosis and will show angulation or translation at the fracture site.

As described, the diagnosis of spondylopelvic dissociation can be made based on plain films; however, in the clinical setting, computed axial tomography with coronal, sagittal, and 3-dimensional reconstructions are the standard of care for diagnosis and operative planning. Computed tomography (CT) cuts of less than 5 mm are mandatory,[15] as are sagittal reformats. The transverse component can easily be missed on the axial sections. Any bilateral sacral fracture should be considered an unstable spondylopelvic dissociation until proven otherwise on the sagittal and coronal reformats. Sacral kyphosis and translation are easily appreciated in the sagittal reformats. In addition, impaction of the cephalad segments into the anterocentral caudal segments produces a characteristic CT finding. Coronal reformats are essential for distinguishing U-, H-, T-, and Y-shaped sacral fractures (**Figs. 4–6**). CT imaging can also give the surgeon insight into the amount of fracture debris in the neural foramina, which can aid in decision-making regarding decompression.[33]

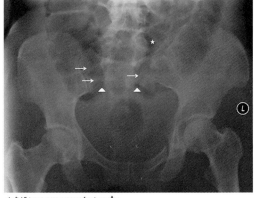

- Left L5 transverse process fracture ★
- Paradoxical inlet view of upper sacrum on AP pelvis plain radiograph ▲
- Upper sacral foraminal line irregularities ⟶

Fig. 3. Anteroposterior radiograph displaying several characteristic findings of spondylopelvic dissociation.

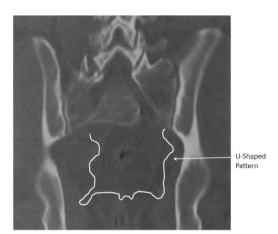

Fig. 4. U-shaped sacral fracture.

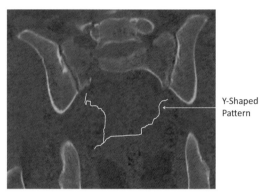

Fig. 6. Y-shaped sacral fracture.

Furthermore, CT is essential for preoperative planning of reduction maneuvers and placement of instrumentation. The utility of magnetic resonance imaging in the setting of acute spondylopelvic dissociation has not been addressed in the literature; however, it may play an important role in assessing the integrity of the posterior ligamentous complex.[1]

TREATMENT

Treatment of spondylopelvic dissociation includes operative and nonoperative options. Definitive treatment goals must take into consideration the systemic injury load and expected duration of activity restriction, especially if bed rest would be required. Nonoperative therapy has been associated with progressive deformity, chronic pain, and the sequelae of recumbency for several months.[1,15] On the other hand, active hemodynamic instability is a contraindication for surgical treatment. These injuries often do not need to be stabilized emergently and, given the systemic stress of the potentially prolonged procedure in a

prone position, the patient should be optimized before surgery.

Nonoperative Management

Lehman and colleagues[1] propose an algorithm for operative versus nonoperative decision-making, which starts by asking if the patient can tolerate surgery. From here it is important to know how long the patient is likely going to be bed bound and how long the patient will be non-weight-bearing bilaterally. If either is more than 3 months, nonoperative management may be considered. Next the surgeon must determine the amount of sacral kyphosis of the fracture. It has been found that if kyphosis is greater than 20°, the deformity likely will progress, resulting in increased instability. In these, patient surgery should be considered. Using these narrow nonoperative criteria, most patients with spondylopelvic dissociation are likely to be managed surgically. These recommendations were proposed based entirely on published case series and expert opinion. There are no prospectively collected randomized data comparing management strategies, likely the result of the rarity with which these injuries are encountered.

Operative Management

Operatively treated patients need to be optimized before surgery. These patients are nearly always polytraumatized and the guidelines of Advanced Trauma Life Support are paramount. Tenets of damage control orthopedics, if applicable and appropriate, should also be considered. As described by Schildhauer and colleagues,[28] indications for urgent/emergent surgery are limited to documented deterioration in neurologic status that correlates with imaging, open injury, and compromised soft tissues related to fracture displacement. Preoperative skeletal traction should be considered in these patients with the goal being to stabilize vertical instability and maintain/improve fracture reduction.[7]

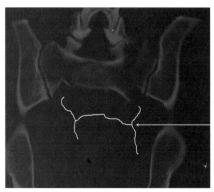

Fig. 5. H-shaped sacral fracture.

This traction can then be used in the operating room for fracture reduction before instrumentation.[28,33–35]

Spondylopelvic dissociation frequently occurs in conjunction with additional pelvic ring trauma.[21] Anterior pelvic ring injuries are typically definitively reconstructed before addressing the spondylopelvic dissociation and may require a staged approach of pelvic external fixation (anterior ring, posterior ring, eg, with C-clamp, or both) followed by open reduction and internal fixation anteriorly and then posteriorly.[28] An anterior internal fixator can also be considered if patient or fracture characteristics make open anterior plating less desirable. Although myriad factors influence the timing of lumbosacropelvic reconstruction, fracture comminution should not be given enough time to begin consolidating before instrumentation. Delayed corrective surgery with osteotomies is exceedingly complex with poor outcomes. The ideal window of appropriate surgical opportunity has been reported to be within 1 to 2 weeks.[28,33]

The evolution of surgical management has been dramatic and greatly influenced by advances in both posterior spinal instrumentation and percutaneous pelvic fixation methods. Before the 1980s, management of transverse sacral fractures was predominantly noninstrumented because adequate operative methods were lacking.[3,4] Fountain and coworkers[5] describe their experience with sacral nerve root decompressions in 1977, while 1979 saw the first report of spinal instrumentation used for fracture reduction and fixation.[6] Fardon[6] describes using a Harrington rod/hook construct and gaining 23° of fracture reduction with distal fixation to the sacral ala immediately adjacent to the vertical components of the sacral fractures. This finding was followed by Roy-Camille and colleagues[7] 6 years later in which they describe lumboiliac plate fixation with bilateral L-shaped plates transfixed by screws into L4 and L5 pedicles and posterior iliac crest. They also discuss their experience with Harrington rod fixation as well as lumbosacral plate fixation in which they were able to control sagittal balance through rigid plate fixation into the ilium via the sacroiliac joint and L4 and L5 pedicles.

The modern era of spondylopelvic fixation surgery commenced in the early to mid 1990s with the description by Käch and Trentz[36] of lumbopelvic distraction spondylodesis in which they performed segmental posterior instrumentation with modern pedicle screw technology from L5 to the ilium. This technique bypasses the sacrum and provides vertical stability. Concerns about rotational stability of the posterior ring prompted Schildhauer and coworkers[37] to modify the lumbopelvic distraction spondylodesis technique. Their construct added horizontal transacral screw

fixation and was termed triangular osteosynthesis. This construct has the benefit of providing translational and rotation stability in the vertical and horizontal planes. A modification to this has been proposed, which substitutes transacral screws for transverse cross-links connecting the vertical rods.[38] Similarly, rotational stability can be added with anterior ring fixation or supplementing a posterior cross-link with iliosacral screws (**Fig. 7**). Although triangular osteosynthesis has gained popularity, less invasive percutaneous methods have developed that may offer reliable alternatives when indicated. First described by Nork and colleagues[15] in 2001, percutaneously guided iliosacral screw osteosynthesis may be used for stabilization of spondylopelvic dissociation in which in situ fixation is acceptable and nerve root decompression is not needed.

When surgical management of spondylopelvic dissociation is being planned, several factors must be addressed. These factors include soft tissue considerations, fracture alignment and reduction, nerve root decompression, and instrumentation techniques.

Soft tissue considerations
Soft tissue quality is of utmost importance when considering posterior midline versus percutaneous incisions and postoperative management.[1] As mentioned, percutaneous iliosacral screw fixation may be an acceptable choice if the lumbopelvic complex is rotationally stable in the sagittal plane. In this situation minimal additional soft tissue trauma is expected and may in fact be well away from the zone of injury. Otherwise triangular osteosynthesis through a more invasive posterior incision is indicated. Both preoperative and postoperative deep pressure injuries related to prolonged immobilization and prominent instrumentation must be aggressively and vigilantly managed. As a part of this, the treating physicians should consider nutritional resuscitation and support in all patients with spondylopelvic dissociation.[26] In addition, the intensive care nursing staff will play a critical role in prevention of preoperative and postoperative preventable soft tissue injury with frequent skin checks and patient rolling.

Fracture alignment and reduction
Kyphosis across the fracture site is commonly seen in these injuries. Subsequently, sagittal plane balance is a critically important consideration and is a well-understood concept in spinal deformity correction surgery and has informed understanding of overall fracture reduction and alignment of spondylopelvic dissociation.[17,24,39] Pelvic incidence (PI) is the gold standard radiographic parameter for

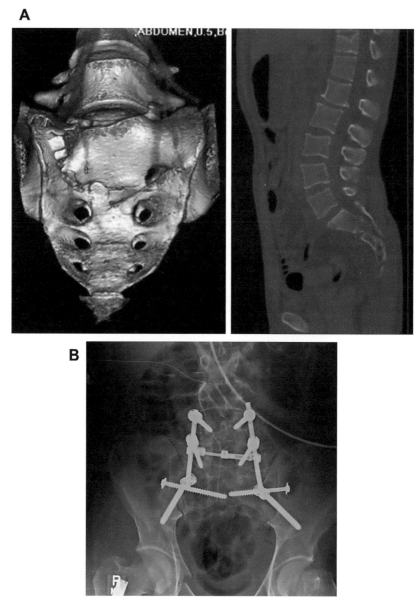

Fig. 7. (*A*) Preoperative images demonstrating a U-shaped sacral fracture with a flexion-posterior translation deformity (Roy-Camille type 2 injury). (*B*) Triangular osteosynthesis. L4-ilium posterior instrumentation supplemented with cross-link and bilateral iliosacral screws.

assessing sagittal plane reduction and understanding the lumbar spine orientation relative to the pelvis. PI is the angle subtended by a line perpendicular to the middle of the S1 endplate and a line from the middle of the S1 endplate to the center of the femoral head on a lateral radiograph. As the superior fracture segment flexes, the PI increases. Normal PI for women is 56 ± 10° and for men is 53 ± 10.6°.[40] Measuring preoperative PI can give the surgeon an objective, intraoperatively measurable goal for reduction (**Fig. 8**). Furthermore, in cases of minimal fracture displacement or

suspected instability an elevated PI alone may be an operative indication.[24] PI is one of the most important preoperative planning considerations. As mentioned, it gives the surgeon an objective correction goal and can be measured intraoperatively with fluoroscopy or CT. Furthermore, the addition of PI to the Roy-Camille fracture type allows for a much more accurate description of the fracture alignment than Roy-Camille type alone.

Once the decision has been made to perform a fracture reduction, numerous techniques may be considered. These techniques include

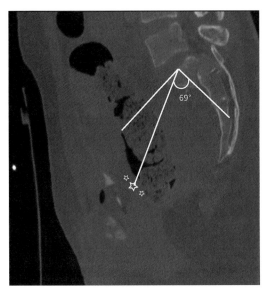

Fig. 8. Increase in (Pelvic incidence) PI after spondylopelvic dissociation. Small stars represent individual femoral head centers.

hyperlordosis positioning with towel bumps,[15] unilateral or bilateral large femoral distractors connected to Schanz pins in the L5 pedicle and ilium,[28] bilateral femoral traction,[28] and even percutaneously placed Schanz pin inserted into the lumbar pedicles and posterior iliac spines used to "joystick" the reduction.[17]

Decompression
The role of nerve root decompression has been extensively debated yet is not well understood.[15,23,28,41] Schildhauer and colleagues[28] reported on 19 consecutive patients who underwent decompression and instrumentation for spondylopelvic dissociation. All 19 patients had incomplete or complete sacral nerve root deficit preoperatively and underwent decompression and instrumentation. Postoperatively 83% had at least some degree of bowel and/or bladder recovery. Of the patients with incomplete preoperative bowel and bladder deficits, 100% regained full sacral nerve root function during the follow-up period, in contrast to the patients with complete preoperative loss of bowel and bladder control in which only 47% regained full control. These results are in-line with several prior small case series in which roughly 70% to 80% of patients regain some element of sacral nerve root function regardless of whether decompression is performed.[28,41,42] However, Ayoub[27] presented his findings of 96.5% of patients with some degree of neurologic recovery after decompression. An important question to consider is whether to decompress a normal functioning nerve

root in which there is fracture debris in its neural foramina. Furthermore, unless there is an acutely declining neurologic status the decompression does not need to be performed urgently and surgical stabilization likely will occur at the same time when safety permits. Another consideration is whether the alignment is in flexion or extension (Roy-Camille type 1 and 2, or 3, respectively), the former being canal shrinking and the latter being canal expanding. In summary, the role of decompression is not well understood; however, the literature would suggest that decompression should be undertaken in all instances in which there is abnormal neurology. Finally, the timing of decompression is likewise not well understood but likely will be dictated by the overall condition of the patient and when major spinal surgery in the prone position is safe.

Instrumentation
The choice of instrumentation is a complex decision process, with several considerations to navigate. The critical component must always be that of operator ability and technical knowhow,[23] which is particularly important in light of the complexity of the injury pattern and the relative rarity with which they present to even busy trauma centers. The next consideration should be directed at the fracture pattern with particular attention to the PI, need for reduction, presence of sacral dysmorphism, and soft tissue insult. The 2 most widely accepted methods of instrumentation are triangular osteosynthesis and iliosacral osteosynthesis. Triangular osteosynthesis requires expertise in spine surgery, is performed through a midline incision in the prone positioning, and is generally considered to impart a larger physiologic load on the patient.[37] Iliosacral osteosynthesis requires expertise in pelvic surgery, may be performed in the prone or supine position, and uses small incisions remote from the posterior midline.[15] In the past, when iliosacral osteosynthesis was used, a closed reduction through patient positioning and skeletal traction was attempted. However, recently, a technique was described in which Schanz pins are percutaneously placed in the lower lumbar pedicles to "joystick" manipulate the fracture into reduction. Once reduced, iliosacral screws are placed to maintain the reduction.[17] With this method, it may be possible to increase significantly the correction that can be achieved with closed methods, which is in contrast to triangular osteosynthesis in which open reduction may be performed through the same incision.

Biomechanically, stabilization of the vertically unstable fractures is significantly better with triangular osteosynthesis compared with iliosacral osteosynthesis. If iliosacral fixation is chosen, transsacral screws should be considered in which fully threaded screws traverse the fracture sites from ilium to ilium. Schildhauer and colleagues[43] showed this through the use of cadaveric specimens with simulated vertically unstable sacral fractures. They investigated fracture behavior through 10,000 cycles of load and their results demonstrated the superiority of triangular osteosynthesis with respect to fracture displacement and catastrophic failure. The mechanical advantages of open osteosynthesis must then be balanced with the soft tissue and physiologic advantages of percutaneous methods.

Surgical outcomes and complications

Functional outcomes in this polytraumatized group of patients are exceedingly hard to assess based on the currently available literature. Reasons for this are several fold and include such factors as poor preoperative documentation of neurologic examination, comorbid injuries, and small case series numbers.[1,19,21] Nerve root decompression is a debated topic with literature suggesting good results both with and without decompression.[28,41,42] Instrumentation is commonly used; however, recent literature out of the military experience in the Middle East suggests several new criteria for a nonoperative approach, including expected bed-bound course of 3 months and bilateral injuries that would result in non-weight-bearing.[1] However, there is no comparative literature of outcomes with operative versus nonoperative management.

Not surprisingly, spondylopelvic dissociation stabilization surgery has an extremely high complication rate and had been reported to be as high as 38.1%.[21] Return to the operating room because of wound complications has been reported to be upward of 25%.[42] The most commonly encountered complications include wound-healing problems, infection, and instrumentation failure. An important and potentially preventable complication is related to prominent iliac instrumentation. Several authors have advocated for recessing or countersinking iliac bolts to prevent soft tissue pressure injury.[26,38] Surgical timing as it relates to soft tissue integrity should be critically assessed to allow for an optimal surgical environment.

SUMMARY

Spondylopelvic dissociation is a highly complex spectrum of diseases seen almost exclusively in the high-energy, polytraumatized patient. Standard radiographic evaluation is exceedingly difficult and advanced imaging in the form of CT scanning is essential for diagnosis and preoperative planning.

Once the diagnosis is made, the complex decision-making of operative or nonoperative treatment must be broached while considering critical patient factors such as soft tissue quality, comorbid injuries, sacral anatomy, surgeon skill. Management options and techniques have evolved over the past 3 decades with the current standards being triangular osteosynthesis and iliosacral screw osteosynthesis. Important future considerations should focus on operative versus nonoperative outcomes, advances in low profile instrumentation, and the role of fracture reduction.

REFERENCES

1. Lehman RA, Kang DG, Bellabarba C. A new classification for complex lumbosacral injuries. Spine J 2012;12(7):612–28.
2. Helgeson MD, Lehman RA, Cooper P, et al. Retrospective review of lumbosacral dissociations in blast injuries. Spine 2011;36(7):E469–75.
3. Purser D. Displaced fracture of the sacrum: report of a case. J Bone Joint Surg Br 1969;51(2):346–7.
4. Bucknill TM, Blackburne JS. Fracture-dislocations of the sacrum. Report of three cases. J Bone Joint Surg Br 1976;58(4):467–70.
5. Fountain SS, Hamilton RD, Jameson RM. Transverse fractures of the sacrum. A report of six cases. J Bone Joint Surg Am 1977;59(4):486–9.
6. Fardon DF. Displaced transverse fracture of the sacrum with nerve root injury: report of a case with successful operative management. J Trauma 1979;19(2):119–22.
7. Roy-Camille R, Saillant G, Gagna G, et al. Transverse fracture of the upper sacrum. Suicidal jumper's fracture. Spine 1985;10(9):838–45.
8. Strange-Vognsen HH, Lebech A. An unusual type of fracture in the upper sacrum. J Orthop Trauma 1991;5(2):200–3.
9. Denis F, Davis S, Comfort T. Sacral fractures: an important problem. Retrospective analysis of 236 cases. Clin Orthop Relat Res 1988;227:67–81.
10. Sabiston CP, Wing PC. Sacral fractures: classification and neurologic implications. J Trauma 1986;26(12):1113–5.
11. Fisher R. Sacral fracture with compression of cauda equina: surgical treatment. J Trauma 1988;28(12):1678–80.
12. Kim MY, Reidy DP, Nolan PC, et al. Transverse sacral fractures: case series and literature review. Can J Surg 2001;44(5):359–63.
13. Robles LA. Transverse sacral fractures. Spine J 2009;9(1):60–9.
14. Ebraheim NA, Biyani A, Salpietro B. Zone III fractures of the sacrum. A case report. Spine (Phila Pa 1976) 1996;21(20):2390–6.
15. Nork SE, Jones CB, Harding SP, et al. Percutaneous stabilization of U-shaped sacral fractures using

iliosacral screws: technique and early results. J Orthop Trauma 2001;15(4):238–46.

16. Vilela MD, Gelfenbeyn M, Bellabarba C. U-shaped sacral fracture and lumbosacral dislocation as a result of a shotgun injury: case report. Neurosurgery 2009;64(1):E193–4.

17. König MA, Seidel U, Heini P, et al. Minimal-invasive percutaneous reduction and transsacral screw fixation for U-shaped fractures. J Spinal Disord Tech 2013;26(1):48–54.

18. Chen HW, Liu GD, Zhao GS, et al. Isolated U-shaped sacral fracture with cauda equina injury. Orthopedics 2011;34(4):316.

19. Yi C, Hak DJ. Traumatic spinopelvic dissociation or U-shaped sacral fracture: a review of the literature. Injury 2012;43(4):402–8.

20. Gribnau AJ, Van Hensbroek PB, Haverlag R, et al. U-shaped sacral fractures: surgical treatment and quality of life. Injury 2009;40(10):1040–8.

21. König MA, Jehan S, Boszczyk AA, et al. Surgical management of U-shaped sacral fractures: a systematic review of current treatment strategies. Eur Spine J 2012;21(5):829–36.

22. Hussin P, Chan CY, Saw LB, et al. U-shaped sacral fracture: an easily missed fracture with high morbidity. A report of two cases. Emerg Med J 2009;26(9):677–8.

23. Hunt N, Jennings A, Smith M. Current management of U-shaped sacral fractures or spino-pelvic dissociation. Injury 2002;33(2):123–6.

24. Hart RA, Badra MI, Madala A, et al. Use of pelvic incidence as a guide to reduction of H-type spinopelvic dissociation injuries. J Orthop Trauma 2007;21(6):369–74.

25. Bents R, France J, Glover J, et al. Traumatic spondylopelvic dissociation: a case report and literature review. Spine 1996;22(11):1276.

26. Vresilovic E, Mehta S, Placide R, et al. Traumatic spondylopelvic dissociation. J Bone Joint Surg Am 2005;87-A(5):1098–103.

27. Ayoub MA. Displaced spinopelvic dissociation with sacral cauda equina syndrome: outcome of surgical decompression with a preliminary management algorithm. Eur Spine J 2012;21(9):1815–25.

28. Schildhauer TA, Bellabarba C, Nork SE, et al. Decompression and lumbopelvic fixation for sacral fracture-dislocations with spino-pelvic dissociation. J Orthop Trauma 2006;20(7):447–57.

29. Kang DG, Cody JP, Lehman RA. Combat-related lumbopelvic dissociation treated with L4 to ilium posterior fusion. Spine J 2012;12(9):860–1.

30. Cody JP, Kang DG, Lehman RA. Combat-related lumbopelvic dissociation treated with percutaneous sacroiliac screw placement. Spine J 2012;12(9):858–9.

31. Schildhauer TA, Chapman JR, Mayo KA. Multisegmental open sacral fracture due to impalement. J Orthop Trauma 2005;19(2):134–9.

32. Gibbons KJ, Soloniuk DS, Razack N. Neurological injury and patterns of sacral fractures. J Neurosurg 1990;72(6):889–93.

33. Sagi HC. Technical aspects and recommended treatment algorithms in triangular osteosynthesis and spinopelvic fixation for vertical shear transforaminal sacral fractures. J Orthop Trauma 2009;23(5):354–60.

34. Gardner MJ, Routt ML. Transiliac-transsacral screws for posterior pelvic stabilization. J Orthop Trauma 2011;25(6):378–84.

35. Mehta S, Auerbach JD, Born CT, et al. Sacral fractures. J Am Acad Orthop Surg 2006;14(12):656–65.

36. Käch K, Trentz O. Distraction spondylodesis of the sacrum in "vertical shear lesions" of the pelvis. Unfallchirurg 1994;97(1):28–38.

37. Schildhauer T, Josten C, Muhr G. Triangular osteosynthesis of vertically unstable sacrum fractures: a new concept allowing early weight-bearing. J Orthop Trauma 1998;20(1):44–51.

38. Mouhsine E, Wettstein M, Schizas C, et al. Modified triangular posterior osteosynthesis of unstable sacrum fracture. Eur Spine J 2006;15(6):857–63.

39. Lazennec JY, Brusson A, Rousseau MA. Hip–spine relations and sagittal balance clinical consequences. Eur Spine J 2011;20(Suppl 5):686–98.

40. Vialle R, Levassor N, Rillardon L, et al. Radiographic analysis of the sagittal alignment and balance of the spine in asymptomatic subjects. J Bone Joint Surg Am 2005;87(2):260–7.

41. Dussa CU, Soni BM. Influence of type of management of transverse sacral fractures on neurological outcome. A case series and review of literature. Spinal Cord 2008;46(9):590–4.

42. Bellabarba C, Schildhauer TA, Vaccaro AR, et al. Complications associated with surgical stabilization of high-grade sacral fracture dislocations with spinopelvic instability. Spine 2006;31(Suppl 11):S80–8.

43. Schildhauer TA, Ledoux WR, Chapman JR, et al. Triangular osteosynthesis and iliosacral screw fixation for unstable sacral fractures: a cadaveric and biomechanical evaluation under cyclic loads. J Orthop Trauma 2003;17(1):22–31.

Pediatrics

Preface
Pediatrics

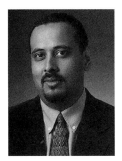

Shital N. Parikh, MD
Editor

Pediatric hip disorders are common and can lead to deleterious outcomes if not recognized or treated in a timely fashion. They can have long-term implications and can potentially lead to end-stage degenerative hip disease. The current issue addresses two of these hip disorders, slipped capital femoral epiphysis (SCFE), which is commonly seen in obese adolescents, and Perthes disease, which is usually encountered during early school years.

With acquisition of new surgical knowledge and skills, the treatment of SCFE continues to evolve. Although in situ fixation and, if needed, subsequent deformity correction continue to be the gold standard of treatment, there is an increasing interest in acute anatomic reduction and stabilization for SCFE. Whether acute repositioning of femoral epiphysis in the setting of unstable SCFE would prevent the disastrous complication of avascular necrosis is still a debatable question. Also, the indications for redirectional osteotomy versus arthroscopic or open treatment of femoroacetabular impingement secondary to residual proximal femoral deformity after healed SCFE continue to be refined. Peck and Herrera-Soto provide a comprehensive review of the current practice and literature to address these controversies related to SCFE.

Perthes disease has baffled surgeons for generations. With limited knowledge pertaining to the etiology of the disease, there is minimal hope to prevent or cure this disease. Treatment and research efforts are rather aimed to prevent the adverse sequelae of the disease. Dr Shah discusses the natural history, prognostic factors, and management of this disease in its active and late stage. Toward the end of the article, Dr Shah discusses the optimal treatment strategies to address adverse sequelae of the disease.

Shital N. Parikh, MD
Pediatric Orthopaedic Sports Medicine
Cincinnati Children's Hospital Medical Center
University of Cincinnati School of Medicine
3333 Burnet Avenue
Cincinnati, OH 45229, USA

E-mail address:
Shital.Parikh@cchmc.org

orthopedic.theclinics.com

Slipped Capital Femoral Epiphysis: What's New?

Kathryn Peck, MD[a], José Herrera-Soto, MD[b],*

KEYWORDS

- Slipped capital femoral epiphysis • Femoroacetabular impingement • In situ fixation
- Surgical hip dislocation

KEY POINTS

- Stabilization of the epiphysis, prevention of slip progression, and avoidance of complications are the desired goals with stabilization of SCFE.
- The controversy on prophylactic fixation derives from the inability to predict which patients will sustain a contralateral slip.
- 32-mm partially threaded and fully threaded screws are valid options for in situ fixation as additional threads in the metaphysis may increase the biomechanical strength.
- The modified Dunn procedure has an incidence of osteonecrosis of up to 26% in the latest series.

INTRODUCTION

Slipped capital femoral epiphysis (SCFE) is the most common hip disorder affecting the adolescent population, with an overall incidence of 10.8 per 100,000.[1] It is characterized by anterosuperior displacement of the metaphysis while the epiphysis remains in the acetabulum. The typical patient afflicted with this disorder is an overweight adolescent boy with groin, thigh, or knee pain, and a limp.[2] Physical examination findings include decreased range of motion (ROM) of the hip, obligate external rotation with hip flexion, and pain with internal rotation. A frog-leg lateral radiograph confirms the diagnosis of SCFE. The etiology of SCFE is usually idiopathic, but can also be seen in patients with endocrine disorders,[3] renal failure,[4] or radiation therapy. Patients with bilateral SCFE initially present with involvement of both hips approximately 50% to 60% of the time.[5] Prophylactic contralateral pinning is controversial among pediatric orthopedic surgeons. SCFE is classified according to 2 methods: the traditional time-based method or the method based on physeal stability and ability to ambulate. The classification system based on physeal stability as described by Loder and colleagues[6] is predictive of prognosis. The unstable SCFE has been reported to have up to 50% incidence of osteonecrosis, compared with a stable SCFE that has nearly 0% incidence of osteonecrosis.[6] Early treatment of SCFE has been supported in the literature as a means to prevent progression of the slip. The classic treatment for stable SCFE has been in situ fixation with a single screw in the center-center position of the epiphysis. Recently, however, there has been a shift in the treatment of SCFE, with the modified Dunn procedure via a surgical hip dislocation emerging as a treatment option for severe SCFE.[7] This method restores the anatomic alignment of the proximal femur and potentially will avoid the sequelae from femoroacetabular impingement. Other treatment options under investigation to improve the outcome of SCFE include computer navigation assistance during in situ

The authors have nothing to disclose.
[a] Hand and Upper Extremity Fellow, The Indiana Hand to Shoulder Center, 8501 Harcourt Road, Indianapolis, IN 46260, USA; [b] Center for Orthopedics, Arnold Palmer Hospital for Children, 1222 S. Orange Avenue, 5th Floor, Orlando, FL 32806, USA
* Corresponding author.
E-mail address: jose.herrera-soto@orhs.org

orthopedic.theclinics.com

fixation, use of an arthrogram during in situ fixation, and arthroscopic-assisted osteoplasty after in situ fixation. The purpose of this article is to present and discuss the latest diagnostic and treatment modalities for SCFE.

PREDICTION OF THE CONTRALATERAL SCFE

Controversy exists among pediatric orthopedic surgeons as to when it is appropriate to stabilize the painless, radiographically normal contralateral hip in a patient who presents with unilateral SCFE.[8] The controversy derives from the inability to predict which patients will sustain a contralateral slip. Those in favor of prophylactic pinning refer to the high incidence of slip in the contralateral hip and the associated devastating complications of osteonecrosis or chondrolysis,[9] in addition to the prevalence of the asymptomatic "silent" slip, resulting in the development of osteoarthritis being reported in up to 40% of cases.[10] The counterargument accounts for the potential surgical complications, including infection, implant complication, chondrolysis, and osteonecrosis.[11]

Riad and colleagues[12] determined that chronologic age was a significant predictor of contralateral slip. In their series of 70 patients with unilateral SCFE, 16 (23%) developed a contralateral SCFE. All girls younger than 10 and boys younger than 12 years developed a contralateral SCFE. Twenty-five percent of girls younger than 12 and 37% of boys younger than 14 years developed a contralateral SCFE (**Fig. 1**). The investigators therefore recommended prophylactic screw fixation in all girls younger than 10 and boys younger than 12 years. To assist in predicting contralateral slips in other patients aside from the very young, 2 methods have recently been reported in the literature: the posterior sloping angle and the modified Oxford bone age score.

POSTERIOR SLOPING ANGLE AS A PREDICTOR OF CONTRALATERAL SCFE

The posterior sloping angle (PSA) of the physis is the angle measured on the Lauenstein axial view between the intersection of the plane of the physis and a line perpendicular to the longitudinal neck-diaphyseal axis (**Fig. 2**).[13] Barrios and colleagues[13] established that the PSA most accurately demonstrates the physeal vertical shear forces that place patients at risk for developing SCFE. In their study of 47 patients, the PSA was found to be 5° in the control group, 12° in patients with unilateral SCFE, and 18° in patients with bilateral SCFE. The investigators concluded that patients presenting with unilateral SCFE demonstrating a PSA of greater than 12° should undergo prophylactic pinning of the contralateral side.

Zenios and colleagues[14] tested the intraobserver and interobserver reliability of PSA, and their study demonstrated a good to excellent reliability of this measurement. Thirteen of their 47 patients in the study group developed a contralateral slip with mean PSA values of 18.8°. Those who did not go on to develop a contralateral hip showed PSA values of 13.9°, and the control group showed a PSA of 3.9°. The investigators concluded that patients with a PSA of greater than 14.5° should undergo prophylactic pinning of the contralateral hip.

Park and colleagues[15] demonstrated the reliability of PSA in a larger series, and also found a difference between sexes, with greater predictability in girls. Phillips and colleagues[16] continued to show the utility of the PSA in the largest study to date in the literature in a predominately Maori population, which is particularly susceptible to SCFE. This study showed that if a PSA of 14° was used as an indication for prophylactic fixation, 83% of contralateral slips would have been prevented and only 21% would have been pinned unnecessarily.

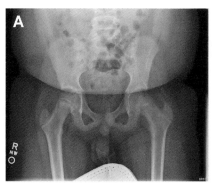 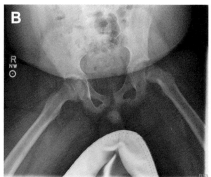

Fig. 1. (*A*) Anteroposterior and frog lateral (*B*) radiograph of a 14-year old boy presented with bilateral slipped capital femoral epiphysis.

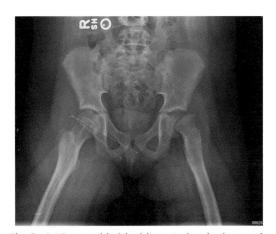

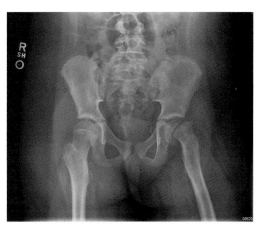

Fig. 2. A 10-year-old girl with posterior sloping angle of 12° as demonstrated on the Lauenstein axial view, a radiograph perpendicular to the hip with the lower extremity in full abduction with the hip flexed at 90°. The posterior sloping angle is the angle formed between the intersection of the plane of the physis and a line perpendicular to the longitudinal neck-diaphyseal axis.

Fig. 3. A 10-year-old girl presented with an unstable SCFE. A modified Oxford score of 18 was calculated for the contralateral side, correlating with a 96% chance of developing a slip of the contralateral side.

Despite the overwhelming evidence showing the PSA of the physis as a predictor of contralateral SCFE, its use has not been widely used in the treatment of SCFE, probably because of lack of awareness or reliability on other proven methods of predicting a future slip.

THE MODIFIED OXFORD BONE AGE SCORE AS A PREDICTOR OF CONTRALATERAL SCFE

The modified Oxford bone age score, as originally described by Stasikelis and colleagues,[17] scored 3 consecutive stages of maturation for 5 radiographic features on anteroposterior pelvic and frog-leg lateral views of patients with idiopathic SCFE. The score ranges from 16 to 26. The lower the number, the younger the patient and the higher the risk of developing a contralateral slip (**Fig. 3**). The iliac apophysis, triradiate cartilage, proximal femoral epiphysis, greater trochanter, and lesser trochanter were the features measured. In their study of 260 patients, 24% of whom developed a contralateral slip, Popejoy and colleagues[18] showed that a modified Oxford bone age score of 16, 17, or 18 had a positive predictive value of developing a contralateral slip of 96% and a negative predictive value of 92%. The study demonstrated that the modified Oxford bone age score and a triradiate score of 1 were significant for prediction of a contralateral slip, with the modified Oxford score being a better indicator (**Fig. 4**). Despite good intraobserver and interobserver reliability, the scoring system of the modified Oxford score is difficult to recall, owing to its basis on

3 continuous stages of maturation. Zide and colleagues[19] modified the scoring system of the 3 stages of maturation to 0, 1, and 2, resulting in an easier ability for clinicians to recall the scoring system and thereby enhancing the use of the modified Oxford score by clinicians. Overall, the modified Oxford score was found to be a reliable predictor of developing a contralateral SCFE.

TREATMENT UPDATES WITH SLIPPED CAPITAL FEMORAL EPIPHYSIS

Stabilization of the epiphysis, prevention of slip progression, and avoidance of complications such as avascular necrosis and chondrolysis are the desired goals with stabilization of SCFE.[6,20] Single in situ screw fixation for stable slips has developed into the most accepted treatment method.[2] Using fluoroscopy, a single cannulated screw is inserted in the center-center position of the epiphysis without progressing closer than 5 mm from the subchondral bone. This method is minimally invasive, not technically demanding, and has a high success rate.[11] In their series, Aronson and Carlson[21] showed excellent to good results in 95% of hips with mild SCFE, 91% of hips with moderate SCFE, and 86% of hips with severe SCFE. Loder and Dietz[22] recently reviewed 65 articles to determine the best evidence for treatment of stable SCFE, which demonstrated that single in situ screw fixation was the best method of treatment.

The type of operating table has also been questioned, as some investigators prefer the radiolucent table to the typically used fracture table. Studies have shown mixed results regarding radiation time, accuracy, and operating time.

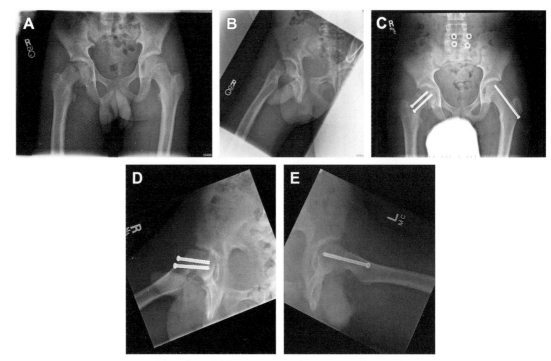

Fig. 4. (*A*) Anteroposterior and frog lateral (*B*) radiograph of a 14-year old male that presented with an unstable SCFE. (*C, D*) He underwent 2-screw fixation of the affected side and prophylactic fixation of the contralateral side (*E*).

With regard to slip progression, Carney and colleagues[23] reviewed 37 children with 46 slips treated with in situ single-screw fixation. In this study, 9 hips demonstrated slip progression, and this progression was linked to the number of threads engaged in the epiphysis. Fewer than 5 screw threads demonstrated progression. Dragoni and colleagues[24] compared 16-mm and 32-mm partially threaded screws and fully threaded screws in a biomechanical porcine model to further evaluate whether the type of screw used during in situ fixation contributed to stability. There was no significant difference detected with the cycles to failure between the different screws used. The 16-mm partially threaded screw did demonstrate a higher frequency of femoral neck fracture, leading the investigators to conclude that both 32-mm partially threaded and fully threaded screws were valid options for in situ fixation, and that the additional threads in the metaphysis may increase the biomechanical strength of the femoral neck.

ARTHROGRAM-ASSISTED IN SITU SCREW FIXATION

Arthrogram-assisted fixation of SCFE has recently been described in the literature as

improving screw placement (**Fig. 5**). Wright and colleagues[25] reported that the screwtip-to-articular surface distance was significantly smaller in the arthrogram-assisted group in comparison with patients in whom only fluoroscopy was used (2.8 mm vs 5.2 mm). The investigators concluded that arthrogram-assisted fixation was an effective method to improve screw

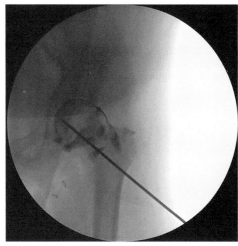

Fig. 5. Arthrogram-assisted in situ fixation of a stable SCFE in an 11-year-old.

placement and visualization, especially when the patient's body habitus makes fluoroscopic imaging difficult to obtain.

COMPUTER NAVIGATION–ASSISTED IN SITU SCREW FIXATION

A prospective comparison of computer-navigated and fluoroscopic-guided in situ fixation of SCFE was also recently reported in the literature. Bono and colleagues[26] reported that screw placement was more accurate with a stealth type of system than with traditional fluoroscopy. The tip to apex distance (6.1 mm vs 8.0 mm) and the distance to the center of the physis (3.2 mm vs 4.9 mm) were significantly improved in the computer-navigation group. An additional 1.9 mm of screw threads engaged the physis in the computer-navigation group; moreover, the computer navigation group achieved the center-center position 91% of the time, compared with only 82% of the time using the traditional fluoroscopic method. The investigators did concede that despite more accurate screw placement, the computer-navigation technology is more expensive not only with respect to monetary cost of the technology but also the need for longer operating-room time. In this study, computer navigation was abandoned because of software problems in one instance and owing to difficulty with navigation and using the fracture table on 3 occasions. The cost-benefit analysis of computer navigation needs to be investigated before this technique is adopted on a routine basis. Although more accurate, the number of pin passes and amount of radiation exposure were similar, and the intraoperative time was longer with the computer-navigated fixation, with no clear benefit to the patient as the differences in accuracy were less than 2 mm.

FEMORAL ACETABULAR IMPINGEMENT AND ACETABULAR MORPHOLOGY IN SCFE

Femoral acetabular impingement (FAI) is a hip disorder caused by abnormal morphology of the proximal femur and acetabulum, resulting in increased hip contact forces with hip motion, most specifically flexion. The increasing hip forces may lead to labral-cartilage injury, and also pain in the adolescent population.[27] FAI is subdivided into 2 types of impingement, pincer impingement and cam impingement, and approximately half of the cases of FAI present with a combination of both types.[27] Pincer impingement is due to overcoverage of the femoral head by the acetabulum.[28] Pincer impingement is typically associated with coxa profunda or acetabular retroversion.[28]

Radiographic findings of pincer impingement include a crossover sign and a posterior wall sign.[29] Cam impingement results from a nonspherical femoral head or femoral retroversion, causing the femoral neck to lever off the anterior rim of that acetabulum.[28]

FAI associated with SCFE can be evaluated clinically, as it forces the patient into obligate external rotation with hip flexion (**Fig. 6**). The Drehmann sign (obligate hip external rotation and abduction with hip flexion) is a clinical finding of patients with SCFE. The obligate hip external rotation and abduction is a way for patients to avoid the pain with motion associated with FAI. Kamegaya and colleagues[30] investigated the relationship between the presence of the Drehmann sign and radiographic evidence of FAI, and found that patients with less remodeling of the proximal femur and higher alpha angles had a much higher rate of presence of the Drehmann sign. The investigators concluded that the presence of the Drehmann sign is highly reliable clinical sign of FAI, and should be taken into account when considering treatment options.

Patients with SCFE are also predisposed to FAI based on the acetabular morphology. Sankar and colleagues[29] evaluated the contralateral hip in patients with unilateral SCFE because of the appearance of overcoverage in the contralateral hip, therefore leading to FAI. The lateral center-edge angle (LCEA) and Tonnis angle are indices of acetabular coverage. In this study, patients with SCFE had an LCEA of 33° and a Tonnis angle of 5°, compared with 20° and 8°, respectively, in controls. Seventy-eight percent of patients with SCFE had a positive crossover sign, and 39% had a posterior wall sign, whereas controls were significantly less measuring 21% and 15%, respectively. The contralateral acetabulum showed significantly more coverage in comparison with age-matched controls, in addition to a higher percentage of retroversion. Both of these features are potential risk factors for developing femoroacetabular impingement.

As discussed previously, in situ fixation has been shown to be a reliable treatment with few complications. However, it has 2 mechanisms through which it can cause FAI. With the epiphysis in the posterior position the screw entry point is typically on the anterior neck, so as to place the screw in the center of the femoral head. A prominent screw head in this location may abut the acetabular rim or impinge on the hip capsule. In addition, the posterior position of the epiphysis that leaves the anterolateral metaphysis exposed causes the prominence to impinge on the acetabular rim.[31] Although this prominence has shown a potential to remodel,[32] significant damage to the

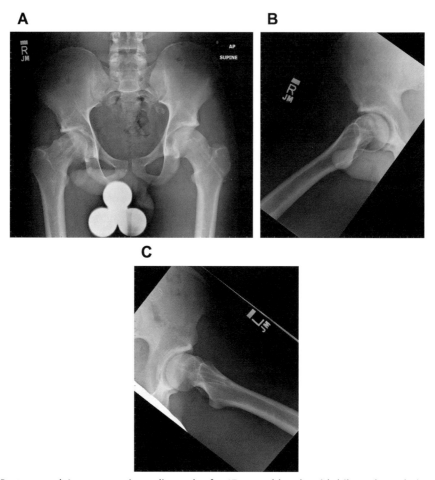

Fig. 6. (A) Post removal Anteroposterior radiograph of a 17-year old male with bilateral cam lesions. He previously underwent in situ fixation for an unstable SCFE of the right hip with 2 cannulated screws (B). (C) Despite prophylactic fixation, the patient demonstrates a left loss of offset on the left hip as well.

labrum and articular cartilage can occur before the remodeling.[33] Because of the damage to the labrum and cartilage, cam impingement has been established as a potential cause of osteoarthritis in patients with SCFE.[31]

Sink and colleagues[34] attempted to classify labral and cartilage damage associated with SCFE by direct observation during surgical dislocation of the hip. Thirty-nine hips were evaluated (8 mild, 20 moderate, and 11 severe), and 33 of 39 hips demonstrated cartilage damage, typically pitting or cleavage deformity, of an average depth of 5 mm. The cartilage damage was most commonly observed in the anterior/superior quadrant, and motion evaluation showed the metaphyseal prominence impinging on the cartilage during flexion. Thirty-four of 39 hips demonstrated labral damage, with the majority having fraying or thinning of the labrum. Thirteen of the 39 hips demonstrated a full-thickness tear or detachment from the acetabulum.

Impingement caused by screw placement on the anterior neck is more commonly seen with the more severely involved slips. Goodwin and colleagues[35] developed a biomechanical study to determine whether placement of the screw perpendicular to the physis produces FAI in a cadaver model. The simulated moderate SCFE showed screw-head impingement on the anterior labrum at 70° of flexion, and the simulated severe SCFE showed impingement at 50° of flexion. Because of the impingement of the screw head onto the anterior labrum, the hip needed to externally rotate to achieve 90° of flexion. Hip ROM, as seen on fluoroscopic views, was used to develop schematics of moderate and severe SCFE. Based on these schematics, a screw starting point lateral to the intertrochanteric line minimizes screw-head impingement. Previously in the literature, screw placement not perpendicular to the physis was reported to delay physeal closure[36] and also allow progression of the slip.[21] Gourineni[37] reviewed

36 hips with stable SCFE and oblique screw insertion. The time to average physeal closure was 5 months, and no complications associated with the screw, such as subtrochanteric fracture or impingement, were encountered. Oblique screw placement is an alternative method of in situ screw fixation that may be more appropriate for slips at high risk of screw-head impingement or subtrochanteric fractures.[37]

SURGICAL MANAGEMENT OF FEMOROACETABULAR IMPINGEMENT ASSOCIATED WITH SCFE

It has been well established in the literature that femoroacetabular impingement is the major mechanism for articular and labral damage in the stable SCFE.[34,38–40] Millis and colleagues[36] advocated that hips with SCFE should be viewed as hips with FAI. The impingement should be treated as a separate issue, and solely treating the physeal instability with in situ fixation is an incomplete treatment because it does not address FAI.[36] The treatment of SCFE is now being thought of as consisting of 2 stages, with the short-term goal of preventing further progression of the slip and the longer-term goal of preventing femoroacetabular impingement, the cause of labral and cartilage damage.

Femoroacetabular impingement leads to decreased hip ROM,[41] hip pain, and an increase in osteoarthritis.[27] Mamisch and colleagues[41] investigated the relationship of proximal femoral morphology and limitations in hip ROM resulting from impingement in 31 hips. The ROM in affected hips with mild slips was comparable with that on the unaffected side. With decreased head-neck offset, SCFE patients showed decreased hip ROM, most significantly in flexion. Moderate slips with decreased head-neck offset showed decreases in ROM similar to those of severe slips. The investigators concluded that in addition to the slip angle, the morphology of the femoral head-neck junction should be considered when evaluating patients for reconstructive surgery.

Traditional methods for addressing impingement from SCFE have included the Southwick,[42] Imhauser,[43] and Dunn[44] osteotomies. A significant risk of avascular necrosis was associated with these techniques. New techniques have recently been reported to address the FAI associated with SCFE, and include arthroscopic femoral neck osteochondroplasty, osteochondroplasty through a limited anterior approach, surgical hip dislocation with femoral neck osteochondroplasty, and flexion intertrochanteric osteotomy. Kuzyk and colleagues[45] recommend hip arthroscopy with osteochondroplasty for patients with mild deformity (slip <15°), and a limited anterior approach for hips with larger slip angles or with a large metaphyseal bump that cannot be fully removed via arthroscopy. For moderate slips, surgical hip dislocation with osteochondroplasty and flexion intertrochanteric osteotomy successfully addresses the alignment abnormalities of the epiphyseal-metaphyseal junction. For more severe slips, a flexion intertrochanteric osteotomy with surgical hip dislocation to restore the anatomy of the proximal femur is recommended.[45]

Leunig and colleagues[46] reported on a series of 3 patients who underwent in situ pinning with arthroscopic osteochondroplasty for slip angles less than 30°. Synovitis with anterolateral labral hyperemia and fraying was present in all 3 hips, and chondromalacia was present adjacent to the damaged labrum. The metaphyseal prominence was resected and the femoral head-neck junction was reshaped. At the time of last follow-up, all patients were free of pain and had returned to full activities without pain. Follow-up in the study was limited to less than 24 months.

Surgical hip dislocation with osteoplasty is evolving as an alternative technique to address the metaphyseal prominence, and is being reported from multiple tertiary centers (**Fig. 7**). Spencer and colleagues[47] reported on 19 patients who underwent surgical hip dislocation with osteoplasty or osteoplasty plus intertrochanteric osteotomy. The Western Ontario and McMaster Osteoarthritis Index (WOMAC) questionnaires and radiographs were assessed. The WOMAC scores were improved postoperatively in both groups (54% in the osteoplasty group and 83% in the osteoplasty plus intertrochanteric osteotomy group). All of the osteotomies healed and no evidence of avascular necrosis was detected. Follow-up was limited to 12 months.

Rebello and colleagues[48] reported on 58 patients with proximal femoral hip deformities of varying etiology who underwent surgical hip dislocation in combination with other techniques to address the proximal femoral anatomy. With regard to deformity in association of SCFE, the WOMAC scores improved postoperatively. The investigators also concluded that surgical dislocation can safely be used to reduce unstable SCFE, which is much less technically difficult than for a stable SCFE because the amount of callus that needs to be resected is less. Three of the 4 cases of osteonecrosis occurred in patients who had undergone femoral neck or intertrochanteric osteotomy for deformities resulting from stable SCFE, and it was concluded that the complication rate was related to the complexity of the reconstruction at the time of dislocation.

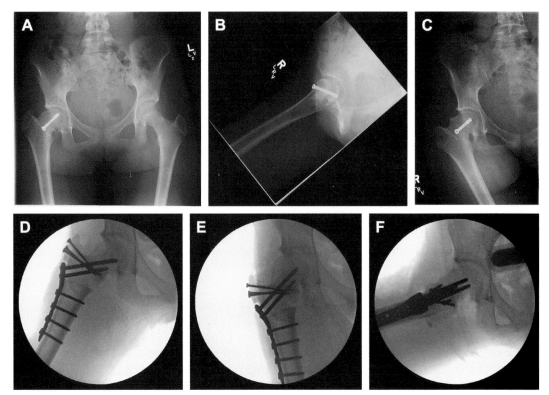

Fig. 7. (*A*) Anteroposterior and frog lateral (*B*) radiograph of a 15-year female who underwent in situ fixation for an stable SCFE presented to the clinic with pain associated with femoroacetabular impingement. (*C*) Maximum adduction radiograph to help plan the amount of valgus needed to correct the femoral head alignment. (*D-F*) The patient underwent correction via a surgical dislocation of the hip with proximal femoral osteotomy to correct the varus and hip retroversion. Labral fraying and cartilage delamination was seen intraoperatively.

Slongo and colleagues[7] reported their results on 23 patients who underwent initial treatment of SCFE with a modified Dunn procedure, which included surgical hip dislocation. Twenty-one (91%) patients had excellent clinical outcomes. Preoperative slip angle of the femoral heal was 47.6°, which was corrected to 4.6°. Postoperative flexion was improved to 107.3° and internal rotation was improved to 37.8°. Two (9%) patients developed severe osteoarthritis and osteonecrosis, and subsequently had a poor outcome. Recently, Sankar and colleagues[49] presented a series from 5 centers, noting satisfactory anatomic correction and excellent clinical results as long as osteonecrosis did not develop. An incidence of osteonecrosis of 26% was reported, and 15% of the patients developed implant failure, all with threaded wires or 4.5-mm screws.

Madan and colleagues[50] reported the outcomes of 28 patients with severe SCFE who underwent treatment with a modified Dunn procedure in combination with a surgical hip dislocation. The lateral slip angle as corrected by mean of 50.9° and the mean modified Harris hip score showed good results. Two (7%) patients developed osteonecrosis

postoperatively. Ziebarth and colleagues[51] reported the outcomes of 40 patients with moderate to severe SCFE who also underwent a modified Dunn procedure in combination with a surgical hip dislocation. Cartilage damage and delamination were observed in 25 of 26 stable SCFEs and 3 of 10 unstable SCFEs. The slip angle was corrected to 4° to 8°. No osteonecrosis was seen at the end of follow-up (1 year and 3 years from 2 different institutions). Delayed union was seen in 3 patients, with subsequent union. One patient required revision surgery for continued signs of impingement. The investigators concluded that subcapital realignment was a safe procedure, and should be used for patients with moderate to severe SCFE and unstable SCFE.

Sink and colleagues[52] reported on a multicenter patient cohort of 334 hips that underwent surgical dislocation in the treatment of various hip disorders causing femoroacetabular impingement for the purpose of evaluating complications associated with the procedure. The overall complication rate was 9%, with the most common complication being heterotopic ossification. There were no cases of osteonecrosis or femoral neck fracture. The only complication reported that might lead to long-term morbidity was a partial resolved sciatic nerve palsy. Six trochanteric non-unions occurred, which resolved with revision open reduction and internal fixation. The investigators concluded that surgical hip dislocation is a safe procedure for addressing femoroacetabular impingement, and has a low complication rate with minimal occurrence of complications resulting in long-term morbidity.

With the development of the novel techniques to address the abnormalities of the proximal femoral anatomy, a low rate of complications was encountered. The complications did include osteonecrosis of the femoral head and a partial resolution of sciatic nerve palsy, both associated with long-term morbidity. Outcomes measures show that patient satisfaction and radiographic measurements improve at short-term follow-up, but long-term outcomes associated with these novel techniques are currently unclear. Long-term outcomes are necessary to completely evaluate these techniques and to assess whether outcomes are improved in comparison with the standard treatment of in situ fixation, which is significantly less demanding and produces with a near null rate of complications associated with long-term morbidity.

REFERENCES

1. Lehmann CL, Arons RR, Loder RT, et al. The epidemiology of slipped capital femoral epiphysis: an update. J Pediatr Orthop 2006;26(3):286–90.
2. Aronsson DD, Loder RT, Breur GJ, et al. Slipped capital femoral epiphysis: current concepts. J Am Acad Orthop Surg 2006;14(12):666–79.
3. Loder RT, Wittenberg B, DeSilva G. Slipped capital femoral epiphysis associated with endocrine disorders. J Pediatr Orthop 1995;15(3):349–56.
4. Loder RT, Hensinger RN. Slipped capital femoral epiphysis associated with renal failure osteodystrophy. J Pediatr Orthop 1997;17(2):205–11.
5. Loder RT, Aronson DD, Greenfield ML. The epidemiology of bilateral slipped capital femoral epiphysis. A study of children in Michigan. J Bone Joint Surg Am 1993;75(8):1141–7.
6. Loder RT, Aronson DD, Greenfield ML, et al. Acute slipped capital femoral epiphysis: the importance of physeal stability. J Bone Joint Surg Am 1993; 75(8):1134–40.
7. Slongo T, Kakaty D, Krause F, et al. Treatment of slipped capital femoral epiphysis with a modified Dunn procedure. J Bone Joint Surg Am 2010; 92(18):2898–908.
8. Kocher MS, Bishop JA, Hresko MT, et al. Prophylactic pinning of the contralateral hip after unilateral slipped capital femoral epiphysis. J Bone Joint Surg Am 2004;86-A(12):2658–65.
9. Yildirim Y, Bautista S, Davidson RS. Chondrolysis, osteonecrosis, and slip severity in patients with subsequent contralateral slipped capital femoral epiphysis. J Bone Joint Surg Am 2008;90(3):485–92.
10. Hagglund G. The contralateral hip in slipped capital femoral epiphysis. J Pediatr Orthop B 1996;5(3): 158–61.
11. Loder RT, et al. Slipped capital femoral epiphysis. Instr Course Lect 2008;57:473–98.
12. Riad J, Bajelidze G, Gabos PG. Bilateral slipped capital femoral epiphysis: predictive factors for contralateral slip. J Pediatr Orthop 2007;27(4): 411–4.
13. Barrios C, Blasco MA, Blasco MC, et al. Posterior sloping angle of the capital femoral physis: a predictor of bilaterality in slipped capital femoral epiphysis. J Pediatr Orthop 2005;25(4):445–9.
14. Zenios M, Ramachandran M, Axt M, et al. Posterior sloping angle of the capital femoral physis: interobserver and intraobserver reliability testing and predictor of bilaterality. J Pediatr Orthop 2007;27(7): 801–4.
15. Park S, Hsu JE, Rendon N, et al. The utility of posterior sloping angle in predicting contralateral slipped capital femoral epiphysis. J Pediatr Orthop 2010;30(7):683–9.
16. Phillips PM, Phadnis J, Willoughby R, et al. Posterior sloping angle as a predictor of contralateral slip in slipped capital femoral epiphysis. J Bone Joint Surg Am 2013;95(2):146–50.
17. Stasikelis PJ, Sullivan CM, Phillips WA, et al. Slipped capital femoral epiphysis. Prediction of contralateral involvement. J Bone Joint Surg Am 1996; 78(8):1149–55.
18. Popejoy D, Emara K, Birch J. Prediction of contralateral slipped capital femoral epiphysis using the modified Oxford bone age score. J Pediatr Orthop 2012;32(3):290–4.
19. Zide JR, Popejoy D, Birch JG. Revised modified Oxford bone score: a simpler system for prediction of contralateral involvement in slipped capital femoral epiphysis. J Pediatr Orthop 2011;31(2): 159–64.
20. Aronsson DD, Loder RT. Treatment of the unstable (acute) slipped capital femoral epiphysis. Clin Orthop Relat Res 1996;(322):99–110.
21. Aronson DD, Carlson WE. Slipped capital femoral epiphysis. A prospective study of fixation with a single screw. J Bone Joint Surg Am 1992;74(6): 810–9.
22. Loder RT, Dietz FR. What is the best evidence for the treatment of slipped capital femoral epiphysis? J Pediatr Orthop 2012;32(Suppl 2):S158–65.
23. Carney BT, Birnbaum P, Minter C. Slip progression after in situ single screw fixation for stable slipped

capital femoral epiphysis. J Pediatr Orthop 2003; 23(5):584–9.

24. Dragoni M, Heiner AD, Costa S, et al. Biomechanical study of 16-mm threaded, 32-mm threaded, and fully threaded SCFE screw fixation. J Pediatr Orthop 2012;32(1):70–4.

25. Wright PB, Ruder J, Herrera-Soto JA, et al. Arthrogram-assisted fixation of slipped capital femoral epiphysis: a CT and radiographic study. J Pediatr Orthop 2012;32(7):693–6.

26. Bono KT, Rubin MD, Jones KC, et al. A prospective comparison of computer-navigated and fluoroscopic-guided in situ fixation of slipped capital femoral epiphysis. J Pediatr Orthop 2013;33(2):128–34.

27. Sink EL, Gralla J, Ryba A, et al. Clinical presentation of femoroacetabular impingement in adolescents. J Pediatr Orthop 2008;28(8):806–11.

28. Parvizi J, Leunig M, Ganz R. Femoroacetabular impingement. J Am Acad Orthop Surg 2007; 15(9):561–70.

29. Sankar WN, Brighton BK, Kim YJ, et al. Acetabular morphology in slipped capital femoral epiphysis. J Pediatr Orthop 2011;31(3):254–8.

30. Kamegaya M, Saisu T, Nakamura J, et al. Drehmann sign and femoro-acetabular impingement in SCFE. J Pediatr Orthop 2011;31(8):853–7.

31. Wenger DR, Kishan S, Pring ME. Impingement and childhood hip disease. J Pediatr Orthop B 2006; 15(4):233–43.

32. Boyer DW, Mickelson MR, Ponseti IV. Slipped capital femoral epiphysis. Long-term follow-up study of one hundred and twenty-one patients. J Bone Joint Surg Am 1981;63(1):85–95.

33. Leunig M, Casillas MM, Hamlet M, et al. Slipped capital femoral epiphysis: early mechanical damage to the acetabular cartilage by a prominent femoral metaphysis. Acta Orthop Scand 2000; 71(4):370–5.

34. Sink EL, Zaltz I, Heare T, et al. Acetabular cartilage and labral damage observed during surgical hip dislocation for stable slipped capital femoral epiphysis. J Pediatr Orthop 2010;30(1):26–30.

35. Goodwin RC, Mahar AT, Oswald TS, et al. Screw head impingement after in situ fixation in moderate and severe slipped capital femoral epiphysis. J Pediatr Orthop 2007;27(3):319–25.

36. Millis MB, Novais EN. In situ fixation for slipped capital femoral epiphysis: perspectives in 2011. J Bone Joint Surg Am 2011;93(Suppl 2):46–51.

37. Gourineni P. Oblique in situ screw fixation of stable slipped capital femoral epiphysis. J Pediatr Orthop 2013;33(2):135–8.

38. Wagner S, Hofstetter W, Chiquet M, et al. Early osteoarthritic changes of human femoral head cartilage subsequent to femoro-acetabular impingement. Osteoarthr Cartil 2003;11(7):508–18.

39. Leunig M, Fraitzl CR, Ganz R. Early damage to the acetabular cartilage in slipped capital femoral epiphysis. Therapeutic consequences. Orthopade 2002;31(9):894–9.

40. Abraham E, Gonzalez MH, Pratap S, et al. Clinical implications of anatomical wear characteristics in slipped capital femoral epiphysis and primary osteoarthritis. J Pediatr Orthop 2007;27(7):788–95.

41. Mamisch TC, Kim YJ, Richolt JA, et al. Femoral morphology due to impingement influences the range of motion in slipped capital femoral epiphysis. Clin Orthop Relat Res 2009;467(3):692–8.

42. Southwick WO. Osteotomy through the lesser trochanter for slipped capital femoral epiphysis. J Bone Joint Surg Am 1967;49(5):807–35.

43. Imhauser G. Late results of Imhauser's osteotomy for slipped capital femoral epiphysis [author's transl.]. Z Orthop Ihre Grenzgeb 1977;115(5): 716–25 [in German].

44. Dunn DM. The treatment of adolescent slipping of the upper femoral epiphysis. J Bone Joint Surg Br 1964;46:621–9.

45. Kuzyk PR, Kim YJ, Millis MB. Surgical management of healed slipped capital femoral epiphysis. J Am Acad Orthop Surg 2011;19(11):667–77.

46. Leunig M, Horowitz K, Manner H, et al. In situ pinning with arthroscopic osteoplasty for mild SCFE: a preliminary technical report. Clin Orthop Relat Res 2010;468(12):3160–7.

47. Spencer S, Millis MB, Kim YJ. Early results of treatment of hip impingement syndrome in slipped capital femoral epiphysis and pistol grip deformity of the femoral head-neck junction using the surgical dislocation technique. J Pediatr Orthop 2006; 26(3):281–5.

48. Rebello G, Spencer S, Millis MB, et al. Surgical dislocation in the management of pediatric and adolescent hip deformity. Clin Orthop Relat Res 2009;467(3):724–31.

49. Sankar WN, Vanderhave KL, Matheney T, et al. The modified Dunn procedure for unstable slipped capital femoral epiphysis: a multicenter perspective. J Bone Joint Surg Am 2013;95(7):585–91.

50. Madan SS, Cooper AP, Davies AG, et al. The treatment of severe slipped capital femoral epiphysis via the Ganz surgical dislocation and anatomical reduction: a prospective study. Bone Joint J 2013;95-B(3):424–9.

51. Ziebarth K, Zilkens C, Spencer S, et al. Capital realignment for moderate and severe SCFE using a modified Dunn procedure. Clin Orthop Relat Res 2009;467(3):704–16.

52. Sink EL, Beaule PE, Sucato D, et al. Multicenter study of complications following surgical dislocation of the hip. J Bone Joint Surg Am 2011; 93(12):1132–6.

Perthes Disease
Evaluation and Management

Hitesh Shah, MS (Orthopaedics), DNB (Orthopaedics)

KEYWORDS

- Perthes disease • Iliac osteotomy • Femoral osteotomy • Containment • Congruent hip

KEY POINTS

- The primary goal of the treatment is to prevent irreversible femoral head deformation, incongruent hip, and femoroacetabular impingement.
- Preventable treatment strategy is more effective in the early stage (before the stage of advanced fragmentation) than in the late stage of the disease. The timing of the surgery is more important than the type of surgery.
- Epiphyseal extrusion is the most important and the only factor that modulates the preventable treatment in early Perthes disease.
- Most younger children can be managed conservatively. Surgical containment is essential for children with late-onset Perthes disease. Normal hip joint movements and absence of hinge abduction are the prerequisites for surgical containment.

INTRODUCTION

Perthes disease is one of the most common pediatric disorders. It is an aseptic, noninflammatory, self-limiting, idiopathic, avascular necrosis of capital femoral epiphysis in a child.[1] One hundred years after its first description, the exact cause of the Perthes disease is not known.[2] The treatment of Perthes disease may be preventive, remedial, or salvageable in nature depending on when the child is diagnosed.

The aim of treating Perthes disease is to prevent secondary degenerative arthritis of the hip in adult life, which can be achieved by preventing the femoral head from getting deformed if the child is diagnosed early, by minimizing the adverse effects of early deformation of the femoral head if it has already occurred, and by salvaging hips with established deformation of the femoral head.[3]

NATURAL HISTORY

Perthes is a self-limiting disorder as blood supply of the femoral head restores to normal within 2 to 4 years' duration following initial avascularization. Single or multiple recurrent episodes of interruption of blood supply of the femoral head occur. Once the blood supply to the femoral head is compromised, a series of events occur within and outside the femoral head. Avascular necrosis of part or all of the epiphysis occurs; the necrotic bone is resorbed by osteoclasts. The weakened trabeculae collapse and the epiphysis fragments. Woven bone is laid down on the periphery of the epiphysis and over a period of time this woven bone is replaced by mature lamellar bone and the epiphysis heals completely. Concomitant changes take place outside the femoral head. Hypertrophy of the synovium, ligamentum teres, and the articular cartilage occurs. These soft tissue changes along with muscle spasm initiate femoral head extrusion that tends to increase progressively. The extruded femoral head, when subjected to stresses that pass across the acetabular margin, lead to irreversible deformation of the femoral head.[4,5] A little remodeling of the femoral head may then occur. Any residual femoral head

The author received no funding support for this paper and as no financial disclosures relevant to this paper.
Pediatric Orthopaedic Services, Department of Orthopaedics, Kasturba Medical College, Manipal University, Manipal 576104, Karnataka, India
E-mail address: hiteshshah12@gmail.com

orthopedic.theclinics.com

deformity and joint incongruity will then persist throughout life.[6,7] Recent evidence has clearly shown that irreversible deformation occurs when the disease has progressed to the late stage of fragmentation or soon after.[1]

Variables that make femoral head deformity worse are femoral head weakening and significant loading. Femoral head weakening correlates with the extent of head involvement.[8] Loading depends on the patient's activity level, type of activities, and weight. Intervention should necessarily precede the onset of irreversible deformation of the femoral head.[9]

EVALUATION OF PROGNOSTIC FACTORS

It is important to know the prognostic factors that affect the final outcome of the disease.

Short-term Prognostic Factors

The factors that determine the shape of the femoral head at the time of healing of the disease include age at onset of the disease, extent of epiphyseal avascularity, extent of epiphyseal collapse, and extent of epiphyseal extrusion.[8,10–12] Early onset of the disease, less than 50% of head involvement, less severe collapse, and the absence of epiphyseal extrusion are good indicators of the outcome. Of these factors, epiphyseal extrusion is the most important and the only factor that can be modulated by treatment.[10]

Long-term Prognostic Factors

The factors that predispose to the development of secondary degenerative arthritis include shape of the femoral head at the time of healing of the disease, congruency between the femur and the acetabulum, and age at onset of Perthes disease.[8,13,14] Degenerative arthritis of the hip joint is correlated with the irregular shape of the femoral head, incongruent hip, and the late onset of the disease.

EVALUATION
Patient Evaluation

The age of onset of symptoms and duration of the disease must be determined. The exact age of onset can guide the planning of the management. Long duration of the disease may cause one to miss the timing for the preventable management strategy. History of passive smoking, which should be evaluated as maternal smoking,[15] at least one smoker living in the child's household,[16] and wood smoke,[17] are associated with increased risk of Perthes disease.

Clinical Evaluation

The child with Perthes disease limps and complains of occasional pain in the groin, hip, or knee. These symptoms may be present for weeks or even months. The examination shows a mild limp and decreased range of motion in abduction and internal rotation. Occasionally, there may be gross limitation of all range of motion. Persistent hip stiffness is a poor prognostic sign. It is essential to gain normal range of motion of the hip joint before considering containment treatment.

Radiological Evaluation

Plain radiographs (anteroposterior [AP] and frog lateral) are useful to diagnose the stage, the extent, and the severity of involvement of the femoral head.[8,10–12] The sequential changes of natural history can be divided into two groups: active disease and healed disease.[1] Disease is considered active when the capital femoral epiphysis looks sclerotic with or without the presence of collapse and reossification. The disease is considered healed when no remnant of avascular bone can be identified on both views. Contrast-enhanced magnetic resonance imaging can clearly define the area of the involvement in the early stage of the disease.[18]

ACTIVE STAGE OF DISEASE
Early Stage of the Disease

The femoral head is subjected to deformation in the late stage of fragmentation or soon after this stage, so the active stage of the disease is divided into the early and late stages. The early stage refers to the stage between early avascular necrosis and early stage of fragmentation. The late stage refers to the stage between late fragmentation and early reossification of capital femoral epiphysis.

Management

The age of the child at onset of symptoms, the extent of involvement, stage of the disease, the range of motion of the hip, and the presence of the extrusion of the femoral head must be considered for treatment in the early stage of the disease.

The age of onset can be further divided into less than 5 years, 5 to 8 years, 8 to 12 years, and more than 12 years (adolescent Perthes disease). Adolescent Perthes disease behaves differently from early onset Perthes disease.[19] Nonsurgical treatment is effective and indicated for children who are young (ie, less than 5 years of age).

Containment

Containment refers to repositioning of the antero-lateral part of the femoral epiphysis within the confines of the acetabulum to protect the femoral head from being subjected to deforming forces. Containment can be done by casting, bracing, femoral, or innominate osteotomy.

Nonsurgical containment

Abduction cast and brace are commonly prescribed for nonsurgical containment. Various types of orthosis (abduction splint) are available. Rich and Schoenecker[20] recently showed excellent results with an A-frame orthosis with hip range of motion. The disadvantages of the brace are that it requires excellent patient compliance and must be worn for a longer period of time. An abduction orthosis is preferred for children less than 5 years who present with extrusion.[3] Abduction orthosis and cast treatment are tedious and psychologically difficult for the older child (ie, more than 5 years old). The author does not use any brace or splint as a definitive treatment for children older than 5 years of age.

Surgical containment

Surgical methods provide prolonged containment to maintain normal femoral head sphericity during revascularization. The age of onset, the presence of epiphyseal extrusion, the extent of the femur head involvement, and the hip range of motion are key variables to be considered before doing containment.

Children with age of onset less than 8 years have a better prognosis than children with age of onset more than 8 years. The prognosis is very good with the age of onset less than 5 years.[6,21] Most children do not require surgical containment. The author considers surgical containment only in those children with extrusion during the course of the disease[3] and noncomplaince with the brace.

For children with age of onset between 5 and 8 years, extrusion is the prime factor for deciding surgical containment. A close follow-up is necessary to monitor extrusion in these children. Surgical containment is indicated for children with more than half of the femoral head involved and the presence of extrusion during the course of the disease.[3] For children with less than 50% head involvement without extrusion, nonoperative treatment with non-weight-bearing is preferred.[3,8] Regular close follow-up of these children is required until the stage of reossification to detect early extrusion.

The natural history of children with the age of onset more than 8 years is not favorable. Surgical containment is more effective than no treatment or brace treatment in older children.[22–24] Surgical containment is preferred, irrespective of the presence of extrusion, because extrusion is inevitable in these children.[1,25] The traditional containment treatment cannot be considered for adolescent Perthes disease (age of onset more than 12 years), because the disease behaves entirely differently from the early onset of the disease.[19]

Normal range of motion of the hip joint is a prerequisite for surgical containment. An abduction cast for 6 weeks is preferred before considering surgical containment in children who fail to regain the normal range of motion after a few days of traction.[25]

Type of osteotomy

No consensus exists about the type of surgical containment (femoral and or innominate osteotomy). Proximal femur varus, varus derotation, varus extension, and varus extension derotation are various proximal femoral osteotomies,[25–29] whereas Salter, triple, and shelf acetabuloplasty are various pelvic osteotomies.[30–32] There is no consensus on the type of femoral or pelvic osteotomy to be considered. The results are essentially the same with both femoral and pelvic containment.[23,33] However, normal range of motion of the hip joint and absence of hinge abduction are essential prerequisites for surgical containment.

The authors prefer subtrochantric femur varus derotation osteotomy for surgical containment. Proximal femur osteotomy is performed with 20° varus, open wedge osteotomy, trochanteric epiphyseodesis, and 20° external rotation. No external immobilization is used following surgery. The implant is kept up until complete healing of the disease. There have been no nonunion or hardware failures.[25]

There are several advantages of femur varus osteotomy: it is technically easy to perform; it is as effective as a pelvic osteotomy; and it does not increase intra-articular pressure. The distinct advantage of this osteotomy is that the duration of the disease can be shortened and it can bypass the stage of fragmentation in one-third of children if it is performed in the stage of avascular necrosis (**Fig. 1**).[34,35]

There are several disadvantages of femur varus osteotomy, such as trochanteric prominence, persistent abductor lurch, shortening, lack of remodeling of varus, worsening of coxa brevis, and the necessity of second surgery for implant removal.[27,36–38] However, open-wedge osteotomy with trochanteric epiphyseodesis has shown minimal shortening and negligible abductor lurch in skeletally mature patients.[39,40]

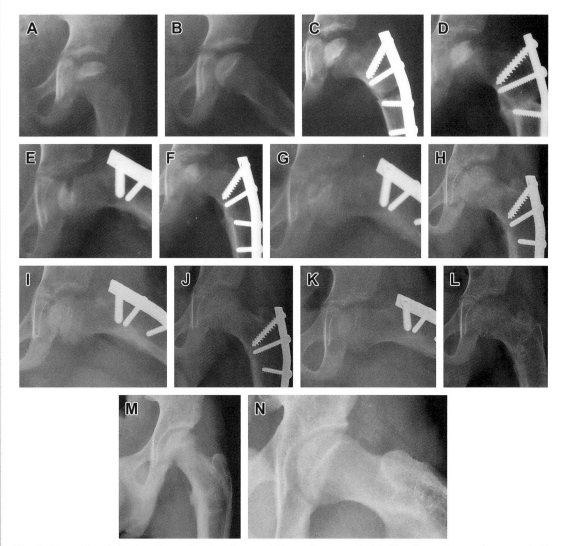

Fig. 1. AP and frog lateral radiographs of an 8-year-old boy who presented in the stage of avascular necrosis (A, B), varus derotation osteotomy was performed (C). Sequential radiographs at 3 months (D, E), 6 months (F, G), 12 months (H, I), and 18 months (J, K) following surgery clearly showed that the stage of fragmentation was bypassed and the disease healed in 20 months (L). Radiographs of the same child at skeletal maturity showed a spherical femoral head, Stulberg class I, sphericity deviation score 0 (M, N).

The pelvic osteotomy is indicated in older children with total head involvement. There are several advantages of pelvic osteotomy, including absence of shortening of the affected limb and no change in the abductor lever arm. No major second surgery is required for implant removal. However, limitations of the pelvic osteotomy are that there is no evidence to suggest that innominate osteotomy alters the natural healing of the disease and overcoverage with triple osteotomy can be associated with pincer impingement.[31]

The use of a combined salter and proximal femoral varus osteotomies has been described for severe disease in older patients, in children more than 10 years of age with severe subluxation, and in those children where either single femur or innominate osteotomy is insufficient to provide adequate containment.[41,42]

Trochanteric Epiphyseodesis

Premature fusion of the capital femoral growth plate occurs in a sizable proportion of older children with Perthes disease,[40] which leads to "greater trochanteric overgrowth" and a Trendelenburg gait. Because premature fusion of the femoral capital growth plate cannot be predicted in Perthes, prophylactic trochanteric epiphyseodesis is recommended at the time of containment surgery in children greater than 7 years of age.[40,43,44] The author routinely combines trochanteric epiphyseodesis with varus derotation femur osteotomy.[40]

Weight-Bearing Status

The absence of weight-bearing in isolation has proved to be ineffective.[45] Kim and colleagues[46] showed that weight-bearing played a significant role in the development of the femoral head deformity and that less flattening occurred with a non-weight-bearing treatment using a large animal model. However, the optimum duration of non-weight-bearing has not been identified. The author thinks prolonged non-weight-bearing up to the late stage of re-ossification prevents the collapse of the soft bone.[47]

Late Stage of the Disease

Children who present late in the late fragmentation stage or reossification stage often have associated femoral head flattening and extrusion. Hinge abduction is common with femur head flattening and extrusion.

Hinge abduction

Hinge abduction is defined as an impingement of the lateral part of the femoral head on the lateral margin of the acetabulum (**Fig. 2**). It can be suspected clinically by sudden deterioration of movements of the hip joint (mainly abduction), out-toeing, or in-toeing gait as a compensatory mechanism.[48] AP radiographs typically show widening of medial joint space in abduction. Dynamic arthrogram can add to the diagnosis of reducible or irreducible hinge abduction; it also helps to decide the best congruent position of the hip joint and the diagnosis of anterior and lateral impingement.[49–51]

Reducible hinge abduction

If the femoral head is centered within the acetabulum without pressing on the lateral margin of the acetabulum, it is considered reducible hinge abduction.[32,51,52] Containment surgery can be performed at this stage; however, the anticipated outcome of the surgery is more modest than the anticipated outcome of the early stage surgery. The odds ratio of obtaining a spherical head at healing is 16.8 times less than if surgery is performed early in the course of the disease.[1] Lateral shelf acetabuloplasty can prevent the subluxation of the femoral head and stimulate lateral acetabular growth.[32,53]

Irreducible hinge abduction

If the femoral head does not center within the acetabulum and the lateral part of the femoral head imposes pressure on the lateral margin of the acetabulum, it is considered irreducible hinge abduction. Various surgeries are described for these noncontainable hips, such as proximal femur valgus osteotomy, articulated hip distraction, shelf and Chiari acetabuloplasty, and femoral head reshaping.

A proximal femur valgus osteotomy is commonly indicated for irreducible hinge abduction to restore joint congruity and to reduce femoroacetabular impingement. It is indicated if the femoral head and acetabulum become congruent when the joint is adducted, but incongruent in a neutral or abducted position.[54] Valgus osteotomy has several advantages: it repositions the abnormal hinge segment away from the acetabulum margin; it increases the weight-bearing surface under acetabulum; it corrects the neck shaft angle; and it increases the abductor muscle length.[51,55]

The degree of valgus should be decided by the maximum joint congruent position in adduction. Valgus osteotomy may also be combined with additional sagittal components. Valgus extension osteotomy is effective when hinge abduction is

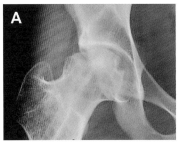
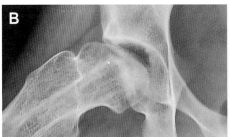

Fig. 2. AP (*A*) and abduction (*B*) radiographs of healed Perthes show typical "hinge abduction". Center of rotation is shifted to the margin of the acetabulum; medial joint space widens medially, and there is increased uncovering of the femoral head.

combined with flexion deformity of the hip with soft anterior hinge that can be contained within the acetabular socket.[56] When the anterior hump is relatively large and noncontainable, extension combination is not indicated because the hump may cause anterior impingement. The rotation component can also be added with valgus, if the hip shows better congruence in internal or external rotation with adduction. If there is an increased subluxation and the hip remains unstable after a valgus osteotomy, a concomitant acetabular procedure (innominate, shelf, or Chiari osteotomy) is necessary to obtain adequate coverage.

Valgus osteotomy is contraindicated in stiff hips. Articulated hip distraction is useful in children who present late with stiff hips and nonreducible hinge abduction.[57] Articulated hip distraction can be combined with soft tissue release.[58] However, the outcome following valgus osteotomy or articulated hip distraction is modest compared with preventable surgery performed in the earlier stage of the disease.[59]

HEALED DISEASE

Once the reossification process is completed, the disease is considered healed, and this can be detected as an absence of sclerosis on plain radiographs. A spherical femoral head with congruent femur and acetabulum relationship at healing are associated with a negligible risk of secondary degenerative arthritis of the hip joint. However, it is difficult to achieve a completely spherical femoral head with congruent hip in all children with healed Perthes disease, and hence, it is important to understand the sequelae of Perthes disease once it has healed.

SEQUELAE OF PERTHES DISEASE
Morphologic Changes in the Femoral Head

If the femoral head is no longer spherical and the contour is irregular, it is known as coxa irregularis. Coxa magna is used for a large femoral head. Because of premature fusion of the capital femoral growth plate, the femoral neck does not grow normally. The short neck with trochanteric overgrowth is known as coxa brevis. All these changes in the proximal femur (coxa irregularis, coxa magna, coxa breva) can predispose to secondary degenerative arthritis of the hip joint.

Failure of Complete Revacularization

Osteochondritis dessicans may develop from failure of complete revacularization, probably due to incomplete revascularization, in a small proportion of patients.

Femoroacetabular Impingement

Abnormal shape of the femoral head and incongruence between the femoral head and the acetabulum may lead to mechanical femoroacetabular impingement (FAI).

Arthritis

Early arthritis may develop, especially in the adolescent form of Perthes disease and is distinct from the late degenerative arthritis that develops in adult life.

Clinical Evaluation of Healed Disease

Groin discomfort may occur with mechanical overload secondary to structural instability, femoroacetabular impingement, or labral disease. Pain and difficulty with upright activities may suggest joint overload or instability. Difficulty with sitting and squatting and limitation of motion may suggest impingement. Discomfort on hip flexion caused by prolong sitting typically indicates FAI. Symptoms like catching and locking indicate intra-articular pathologic abnormality. It is also important to detect knee valgus because of the natural consequence of the disease or following proximal femur varus osteotomy.[60]

The range of motion is restricted in the presence of intra-articular and extra-articular impingement.[61] Hip abductor strength, knee alignment, limb length discrepancy, limitation of range of motion, Tredelenburg sign, impingement sign, and instability test are essential during physical examination to detect early consequences of healed Perthes.

Radiological Evaluation of Healed Disease

Standing plain radiographs (AP and frog lateral) are initially useful for the evaluation of healed Perthes disease. Size and shape of the femoral head, neck shaft angle, position of the greater trochanter in relation to center and articular margin of the femoral head, lateralization of the greater trochanter, congruency of the hip joint, subluxation, and acetabulum retroversion must be clearly defined on plain radiographs. A false profile view is indicated in suspected FAI to detect overcoverage. Computed tomographic scan can better define and quantify femur and acetabulum version and proximal femur deformity in suspected case of FAI.[62] Magnetic resonance imaging delineates articular cartilage, physis, and labral pathologic abnormality better than any other modality.[63] Delayed gadolinium-enhanced magnetic resonance imaging is useful in evaluating integrity of articular cartilage.[64] Arthrogram (intraoperative or magnetic resonance arthrogram) may be useful during surgery to identify the dynamic relationship of the femur and the acetabulum.

Management of Sequelae

Coxa brevis

The distal and lateral transfer of the greater trochanter improves the mechanics of the joint, abolishes the Tredelenburg gait, and reduces stress on the hip.[65] Femur neck lengthening described by Hasler and Morscher is indicated to correct coxa vara, trochanteric overgrowth with correction of limb length discrepancy.[66,67] Coxa brevis correction can also be combined with other procedures for intra-articular pathologic abnormality by safe surgical dislocation of the hip.[68]

Coxa magna

Shelf acetabuloplasty is indicated to improve coverage of the enlarged spherical or ovoid femoral head and may reduce stresses on the hip.

Coxa planna

Femoral head reduction osteotomy may be indicated in grossly deformed nonspherical incongruent hip.[69] Earlier results of the surgery look satisfactory; however, long-term results of these surgeries are yet to be determined. The exact indication of the surgery is not defined.

Osteochondritis dessicans

The optimum treatment for osteochondritis dessicans has not yet been defined. The primary treatment should be conservative. If the fragment becomes loose and interferes with the mechanics of the hip, excision of the fragment may be indicated.[70]

FAI

The transtrochanteric surgical hip dislocation provides complete access to the hip joint and offers the potential for comprehensive correction of severe proximal femur deformities and chondrolabral disease. Arthrogram may be useful to assess the position of hip impingement and guide surgical planning. Safe surgical dislocation and femoral head neck osteochondroplasty are useful for the typical aspherical head with cam or mixed-type impingement by using a spherical femoral head template to guide the resection. In a few cases, whereby the central head is devoid of articular cartilage, central head resection of Ganz and colleagues[69] may be indicated. The femoral head neck osteochondroplasty with relative neck lengthening relieves most impingement. If hip abduction is still limited, and the joint is incongruent in the neutral position, then valgus osteotomy of proximal femur can be combined. Acetabular procedure is indicated if the hip

remains unstable or incongruent after a femoral procedure. If the chondro-labral junction is unstable and there is a significant pincer component, then acetabular rim resection may be required with repair of the labrum.[71]

Arthritis

The salvage operations, including surface replacement,[72] total joint arthroplasty,[73] or arthrodesis,[19] may be needed to deal with arthritis that develops in childhood or adolescence.

In short, joint-preserving surgery with specific treatment of individual structural abnormalities is indicated in symptomatic healed Perthes patients.[74] Restoration of near normal proximal femur morphology results in marked improvement in functional outcomes. Short-term results of joint reconstruction of healed Perthes look promising. However, long-term results remain to be determined.

EVALUATION OF THE OUTCOME AT SKELETAL MATURITY

There are several measures described in the literature to evaluate the outcomes following healed Perthes disease (shape of femur head, congruency of the hip joint). A precise definition of the method of evaluation is necessary to compare the results from various treatment modalities.

Mose[13] describes various types of shape of femoral head with the help of a template in a plain radiograph at skeletal maturity in healed Perthes disease. He categorizes the shape of the femoral head into 3 categories: spherical, fair, and irregular.

Stulberg and colleagues[14] describe the natural history of Perthes disease in long-term follow-up. The sphericity of the femur head and congruency between the femur and acetabulum are important variables that influence the long-term condition of the hip joint. They divide the hips into 5 classes with 3 types of congruency: spherical congruency (class I and II); aspherical congruency (class III and IV); and aspherical incongruency (class V) (**Fig. 3**). Degenerative arthritis does not develop with class I and II hips, whereas severe arthritis develops at less than 50 years of age with class V hips.

A new reliable quantitative measure (sphericity deviation score) of the outcome of Perthes disease has been devised. It will be useful to reduce the sample size if a level I study in Perthes disease is planned.[75]

FUTURE OF PERTHES

Bisphosphonate decreases femoral head deformity in animal model of Perthes disease by

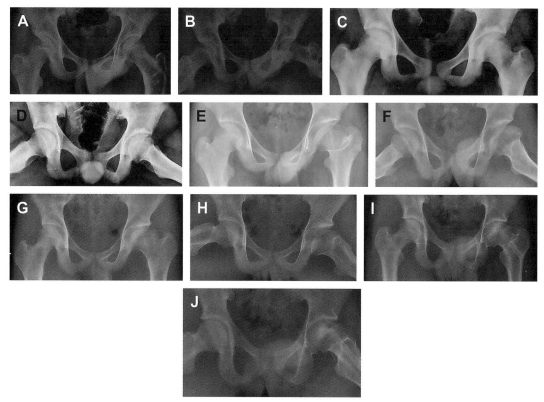

Fig. 3. Various examples of Stulberg outcome at skeletal maturity. (*A, B*) Class I, spherical congruency with normal size of femoral head, neck, and acetabulum. (*C, D*) Class II, spherical congruency with mild coxa magna and coxa breva. (*E, F*) Class III, aspherical congruency with ovoid femoral head (not flat), coxa magna, coxa breva, and persistent acetabular dysplasia. (*G, H*) Class IV, aspherical congruency with flat femoral head, coxa magna, coxa breva, and persistent acetabular dysplasia. (*I, J*) Class V, aspherical incongruency with flat irregular femoral head, mild coxa magna, and normal acetabulum (no acetabulum dysplasia).

decreasing bone resorption. It delays resorption of necrotic bone, which may allow more time for revascularization to occur before strength failure. Although the role of bisphosphonate has been proven in an animal model, there are no clinical studies to prove the optimum dose, site, and duration to recommend the use of bisphosphonate in clinical practice. The future may provide pharmacologic or biological treatment options that will speed up the healing process by decreasing bone resorption and stimulating bone formation.[76]

REFERENCES

1. Joseph B, Varghese G, Mulpuri K, et al. Natural evolution of Perthes disease: a study of 610 children under 12 years of age at disease onset. J Pediatr Orthop 2003;23:590–600.
2. Price CT, Joseph B. Legg-Calve-Perthes disease. Orthop Clin North Am 2011;42:xi.
3. Joseph B, Price CT. Consensus statements on the management of Perthes disease. Orthop Clin North Am 2011;42:437–40.
4. Axer A, Schiller MG. The pathogenesis of the early deformity of the capital femoral epiphysis in Legg-Calve-Perthes syndrome (L.C.P.S.). An arthrographic study. Clin Orthop Relat Res 1972;84:106–15.
5. Herring JA, Williams JJ, Neustadt JN, et al. Evolution of femoral head deformity during the healing phase of Legg-Calve-Perthes disease. J Pediatr Orthop 1993;13:41–5.
6. Ippolito E, Tudisco C, Farsetti P. The long-term prognosis of unilateral Perthes' disease. J Bone Joint Surg Br 1987;69:243–50.
7. Yrjonen T. Prognosis in Perthes' disease after non-containment treatment. 106 hips followed for 28-47 years. Acta Orthop Scand 1992;63:523–6.
8. Catterall A. The natural history of Perthes' disease. J Bone Joint Surg Br 1971;53:37–53.
9. Joseph B, Price CT. Principles of containment treatment aimed at preventing femoral head deformation in Perthes disease. Orthop Clin North Am 2011;42:317–27, vi.
10. Green NE, Beauchamp RD, Griffin PP. Epiphyseal extrusion as a prognostic index in Legg-Calve-Perthes disease. J Bone Joint Surg Am 1981;63:900–5.

11. Herring JA, Neustadt JB, Williams JJ, et al. The lateral pillar classification of Legg-Calve-Perthes disease. J Pediatr Orthop 1992;12:143–50.

12. Salter RB, Thompson GH. Legg-Calve-Perthes disease. The prognostic significance of the subchondral fracture and a two-group classification of the femoral head involvement. J Bone Joint Surg Am 1984;66:479–89.

13. Mose K. Methods of measuring in Legg-Calve-Perthes disease with special regard to the prognosis. Clin Orthop Relat Res 1980;(150):103–9.

14. Stulberg SD, Cooperman DR, Wallensten R. The natural history of Legg-Calve-Perthes disease. J Bone Joint Surg Am 1981;63:1095–108.

15. Bahmanyar S, Montgomery SM, Weiss RJ, et al. Maternal smoking during pregnancy, other prenatal and perinatal factors, and the risk of Legg-Calve-Perthes disease. Pediatrics 2008;122: e459–64.

16. Gordon JE, Schoenecker PL, Osland JD, et al. Smoking and socio-economic status in the etiology and severity of Legg-Calve-Perthes' disease. J Pediatr Orthop B 2004;13:367–70.

17. Daniel AB, Shah H, Kamath A, et al. Environmental tobacco and wood smoke increase the risk of Legg-Calve-Perthes disease. Clin Orthop Relat Res 2012;470:2369–75.

18. Kim HK, Kaste S, Dempsey M, et al. A comparison of non-contrast and contrast-enhanced MRI in the initial stage of Legg-Calve-Perthes disease. Pediatr Radiol 2013;43(9):1166–73.

19. Joseph B, Mulpuri K, Varghese G. Perthes' disease in the adolescent. J Bone Joint Surg Br 2001;83: 715–20.

20. Rich MM, Schoenecker PL. Management of Legg-Calve-Perthes disease using an A-frame orthosis and hip range of motion: a 25-year experience. J Pediatr Orthop 2013;33:112–9.

21. Salter RB. The present status of surgical treatment for Legg-Perthes disease. J Bone Joint Surg Am 1984;66:961–6.

22. Herring JA. Legg-Calve-Perthes disease at 100: a review of evidence-based treatment. J Pediatr Orthop 2011;31:S137–40.

23. Herring JA, Kim HT, Browne R. Legg-Calve-Perthes disease. Part II: prospective multicenter study of the effect of treatment on outcome. J Bone Joint Surg Am 2004;86-A:2121–34.

24. Wiig O, Terjesen T, Svenningsen S. Prognostic factors and outcome of treatment in Perthes' disease: a prospective study of 368 patients with five-year follow-up. J Bone Joint Surg Br 2008; 90:1364–71.

25. Joseph B, Srinivas G, Thomas R. Management of Perthes disease of late onset in southern India. The evaluation of a surgical method. J Bone Joint Surg Br 1996;78:625–30.

26. Axer A, Gershuni DH, Hendel D, et al. Indications for femoral osteotomy in Legg-Calve-Perthes disease. Clin Orthop Relat Res 1980;(150):78–87.

27. Kitakoji T, Hattori T, Kitoh H, et al. Which is a better method for Perthes' disease: femoral varus or Salter osteotomy? Clin Orthop Relat Res 2005;(430):163–70.

28. Ito H, Minami A, Suzuki K, et al. Three-dimensionally corrective external fixator system for proximal femoral osteotomy. J Pediatr Orthop 2001;21:652–6.

29. Menelaus MB. Lessons learned in the management of Legg-Calve-Perthes disease. Clin Orthop Relat Res 1986;(209):41–8.

30. Saran N, Varghese R, Mulpuri K. Do femoral or salter innominate osteotomies improve femoral head sphericity in Legg-Calve-Perthes disease? A meta-analysis. Clin Orthop Relat Res 2012;470: 2383–93.

31. Hosalkar H, Munhoz da Cunha AL, Baldwin K, et al. Triple innominate osteotomy for Legg-Calve-Perthes disease in children: does the lateral coverage change with time? Clin Orthop Relat Res 2012;470:2402–10.

32. Yoo WJ, Choi IH, Cho TJ, et al. Shelf acetabuloplasty for children with Perthes' disease and reducible subluxation of the hip: prognostic factors related to hip remodelling. J Bone Joint Surg Br 2009;91:1383–7.

33. Sponseller PD, Desai SS, Millis MB. Comparison of femoral and innominate osteotomies for the treatment of Legg-Calve-Perthes disease. J Bone Joint Surg Am 1988;70:1131–9.

34. Joseph B, Rao N, Mulpuri K, et al. How does a femoral varus osteotomy alter the natural evolution of Perthes' disease? J Pediatr Orthop B 2005;14:10–5.

35. Wichlacz W, Sotirow B, Sionek A, et al. Surgical outcome for children in the early phase of Perthes' disease. Ortop Traumatol Rehabil 2004;6:712–7.

36. Leitch JM, Paterson DC, Foster BK. Growth disturbance in Legg-Calve-Perthes disease and the consequences of surgical treatment. Clin Orthop Relat Res 1991;(262):178–84.

37. Mirovsky Y, Axer A, Hendel D. Residual shortening after osteotomy for Perthes' disease. A comparative study. J Bone Joint Surg Br 1984; 66:184–8.

38. Bowen JR, Schreiber FC, Foster BK, et al. Premature femoral neck physeal closure in Perthes' disease. Clin Orthop Relat Res 1982;(171):24–9.

39. Shah H, Siddesh ND, Joseph B. To what extent does remodeling of the proximal femur and the acetabulum occur between disease healing and skeletal maturity in Perthes disease? A radiological study. J Pediatr Orthop 2008;28:711–6.

40. Shah H, Siddesh ND, Joseph B, et al. Effect of prophylactic trochanteric epiphyseodesis in older

children with Perthes' disease. J Pediatr Orthop 2009;29:889–95.

41. Javid M, Wedge JH. Radiographic results of combined Salter innominate and femoral osteotomy in Legg-Calve-Perthes disease in older children. J Child Orthop 2009;3:229–34.

42. Chakirgil GS, Isitman AT, Ceten I. Double osteotomy operation in the surgical treatment of coxa plana disease. Orthopedics 1985;8:1495–504.

43. Kitoh H, Kaneko H, Mishima K, et al. Prognostic factors for trochanteric overgrowth after containment treatment in Legg-Calve-Perthes disease. J Pediatr Orthop B 2013;22(5):432–6.

44. Matan AJ, Stevens PM, Smith JT, et al. Combination trochanteric arrest and intertrochanteric osteotomy for Perthes' disease. J Pediatr Orthop 1996;16:10–4.

45. Nomura T, Terayama K, Watanabe S. Perthes' disease: a comparison between two methods of treatment, Thomas' splint and femoral osteotomy. Arch Orthop Trauma Surg 1980;97:135–40.

46. Kim HK, Aruwajoye O, Stetler J, et al. Effects of non-weight-bearing on the immature femoral head following ischemic osteonecrosis: an experimental investigation in immature pigs. J Bone Joint Surg Am 2012;94:2228–37.

47. Tercier S, Shah H, Siddesh ND, et al. Does proximal femoral varus osteotomy in Legg-Calvé-Perthes disease predispose to angular mal-alignment of the knee? A clinical and radiographic study at skeletal maturity. J Child Orthop 2013;7:205–11.

48. Yoo WJ, Choi IH, Cho TJ, et al. Out-toeing and in-toeing in patients with Perthes disease: role of the femoral hump. J Pediatr Orthop 2008;28:717–22.

49. Nakamura J, Kamegaya M, Saisu T, et al. Hip arthrography under general anesthesia to refine the definition of hinge abduction in Legg-Calve-Perthes disease. J Pediatr Orthop 2008;28:614–8.

50. Snow SW, Keret D, Scarangella S, et al. Anterior impingement of the femoral head: a late phenomenon of Legg-Calve-Perthes' disease. J Pediatr Orthop 1993;13:286–9.

51. Yoo WJ, Choi IH, Chung CY, et al. Valgus femoral osteotomy for hinge abduction in Perthes' disease. Decision-making and outcomes. J Bone Joint Surg Br 2004;86:726–30.

52. Daly K, Bruce C, Catterall A. Lateral shelf acetabuloplasty in Perthes' disease. A review of the end of growth. J Bone Joint Surg Br 1999;81:380–4.

53. Domzalski ME, Glutting J, Bowen JR, et al. Lateral acetabular growth stimulation following a labral support procedure in Legg-Calve-Perthes disease. J Bone Joint Surg Am 2006;88:1458–66.

54. Choi IH, Yoo WJ, Cho TJ, et al. The role of valgus osteotomy in LCPD. J Pediatr Orthop 2011;31: S217–22.

55. Myers GJ, Mathur K, O'Hara J. Valgus osteotomy: a solution for late presentation of hinge abduction in Legg-Calve-Perthes disease. J Pediatr Orthop 2008;28:169–72.

56. Bankes MJ, Catterall A, Hashemi-Nejad A. Valgus extension osteotomy for 'hinge abduction' in Perthes' disease. Results at maturity and factors influencing the radiological outcome. J Bone Joint Surg Br 2000;82:548–54.

57. Sudesh P, Bali K, Mootha AK, et al. Arthrodiastasis and surgical containment in severe late-onset Perthes disease: an analysis of 14 patients. Acta Orthop Belg 2010;76:329–34.

58. Segev E. Treatment of severe late onset Perthes' disease with soft tissue release and articulated hip distraction. J Pediatr Orthop B 2004;13:345.

59. Kim HT, Gu JK, Bae SH, et al. Does valgus femoral osteotomy improve femoral head roundness in severe Legg-Calve-Perthes disease? Clin Orthop Relat Res 2013;471:1021–7.

60. Glard Y, Katchburian MV, Jacquemier M, et al. Genu valgum in Legg-Calve-Perthes disease treated with femoral varus osteotomy. Clin Orthop Relat Res 2009;467:1587–90.

61. Tannast M, Hanke M, Ecker TM, et al. LCPD: reduced range of motion resulting from extra- and intraarticular impingement. Clin Orthop Relat Res 2012;470:2431–40.

62. Beaule PE, Zaragoza E, Motamedi K, et al. Three-dimensional computed tomography of the hip in the assessment of femoroacetabular impingement. J Orthop Res 2005;23:1286–92.

63. Carvalho Maranho DA, Nogueira-Barbosa MH, Zamarioli A, et al. MRI abnormalities of the acetabular labrum and articular cartilage are common in healed legg-calve-perthes disease with residual deformities of the hip. J Bone Joint Surg Am 2013;95:256–65.

64. Zilkens C, Holstein A, Bittersohl B, et al. Delayed gadolinium-enhanced magnetic resonance imaging of cartilage in the long-term follow-up after Perthes disease. J Pediatr Orthop 2010;30:147–53.

65. Macnicol MF, Makris D. Distal transfer of the greater trochanter. J Bone Joint Surg Br 1991;73:838–41.

66. Hasler CC, Morscher EW. Femoral neck lengthening osteotomy after growth disturbance of the proximal femur. J Pediatr Orthop B 1999;8:271–5.

67. Standard SC. Treatment of coxa brevis. Orthop Clin North Am 2011;42:373–87, vii.

68. Anderson LA, Erickson JA, Severson EP, et al. Sequelae of Perthes disease: treatment with surgical hip dislocation and relative femoral neck lengthening. J Pediatr Orthop 2010;30:758–66.

69. Ganz R, Horowitz K, Leunig M. Algorithm for femoral and periacetabular osteotomies in complex hip deformities. Clin Orthop Relat Res 2010; 468:3168–80.

70. Rowe SM, Moon ES, Yoon TR, et al. Fate of the osteochondral fragments in osteochondritis dissecans after Legg-Calve-Perthes' disease. J Bone Joint Surg Br 2002;84:1025–9.

71. Peters CL, Schabel K, Anderson L, et al. Open treatment of femoroacetabular impingement is associated with clinical improvement and low complication rate at short-term followup. Clin Orthop Relat Res 2010;468:504–10.

72. Boyd HS, Ulrich SD, Seyler TM, et al. Resurfacing for Perthes disease: an alternative to standard hip arthroplasty. Clin Orthop Relat Res 2007;465:80–5.

73. Thillemann TM, Pedersen AB, Johnsen SP, et al. Implant survival after primary total hip arthroplasty due to childhood hip disorders: results from the Danish Hip Arthroplasty Registry. Acta Orthop 2008;79:769–76.

74. Albers CE, Steppacher SD, Ganz R, et al. Joint-preserving surgery improves pain, range of motion, and abductor strength after Legg-Calve-Perthes disease. Clin Orthop Relat Res 2012;470:2450–61.

75. Shah H, Siddesh ND, Pai H, et al. Quantitative measures for evaluating the radiographic outcome of Legg-Calve-Perthes disease. J Bone Joint Surg Am 2013;95:354–61.

76. Kim HK. Pathophysiology and new strategies for the treatment of Legg-Calve-Perthes disease. J Bone Joint Surg Am 2012;94:659–69.

Oncology

Preface: Wound Complications and Metastases, Insights from Orthopedic Oncology

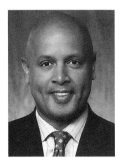

Felasfa M. Wodajo, MD
Editor

In the oncology section of this issue of *Orthopedic Clinics of North America*, we explore two topics commonly encountered by orthopedic surgeons - wound complications and bone metastases, where the experience of orthopedic oncologists might be particularly helpful.

Due to the combination of large incisions and large tissue defects, sometimes in the setting of previous radiation therapy, orthopedic oncologists necessarily become adept in the management and healing of complex wounds. In "Management of Open Wounds: Lessons from Orthopedic Oncology," Dr Herrick Siegel shares his experience and his techniques, including negative pressure wound dressings, silver-coated dressings, and hyperbaric oxygen therapy while drawing on literature published by others and his group at the University of Alabama at Birmingham Medical Center, where he is Professor of Surgery and Section Head of Orthopaedic Oncology.

In "The Practicing Orthopedic Surgeon's Guide to Managing Long Bone Metastases," Dr Felix Cheung assembles a clear and understandable guide for surgical decision-making in the setting of known or suspected bone metastases,

incorporating stratification schemes such as the Mirel score, along with anatomy-specific case vignettes. Dr Cheung is currently Associate Professor and Chief, Orthopaedic Oncology at Marshall University, Joan C. Edwards School of Medicine in Huntington, West Virginia. Patients with metastatic bone lesions can be challenging for practicing orthopedic surgeons; hopefully this article can make these consultations simpler.

Felasfa M. Wodajo, MD
Musculoskeletal Tumor Surgery
Virginia Hospital Center
Arlington, VA 22205, USA

Orthopedic Surgery
Georgetown University Hospital
Washington, DC, USA

Orthopedic Surgery
VCU School of Medicine
Inova Campus
Falls Church, VA, USA

E-mail address:
wodajo@tumors.md

Orthop Clin N Am 45 (2014) xix
http://dx.doi.org/10.1016/j.ocl.2013.10.002
0030-5898/14/$ – see front matter © 2014 Elsevier Inc. All rights reserved.

Management of Open Wounds
Lessons from Orthopedic Oncology

Herrick J. Siegel, MD

KEYWORDS

- Sarcoma • Wound complications • Hyperbaric oxygen treatment • Silver dressings

KEY POINTS

- Using a multifactorial approach to the management of massive wounds will likely facilitate healing of massive, complex wounds as a result of tumor, trauma, and/or infection.
- The combination of hyperbaric oxygen treatment, wound vacuum-assisted closure therapy, and silver dressings has great potential and seem to reduce the morbidity and cost of wound management.
- Future randomized studies are needed to understand the impact of each modality better.
- Studying sarcoma patients and the complexity associated with wound care due to soft tissue loss, prior radiation exposure, and immunosuppression from chemotoxicity will likely lead to future improvements and the development of other modalities to improve wound care.

WOUND COMPLICATIONS IN SARCOMA TREATMENT

For most sarcoma patients, limb-sparing surgery is the standard of care. Functional outcome and quality of life are major concerns when considering surgical resection and reconstruction. Radiation is an effective means to reduce the incidence of recurrence, particularly in high-grade soft tissue sarcoma. However the combination of radiation and limb salvage has created its own set of complications in terms of wound complications.[1,2] Pelvic and sacral resections remain a challenge for wound complications. A multidisciplinary approach is often needed to optimize the patient's functional and cancer outcome successfully; early referral to a sarcoma center is important (**Fig. 1**).

Radiation administered in conjunction with surgery is designed to eliminate tumor recurrence from close or positive margins. The risk of recurrence can be substantially reduced by using either preoperative or postoperative adjuvant radiation. The traditional method of providing radiation in conjunction with surgery is to begin radiation after surgery once postoperative wound healing is completed. However, postoperative radiation treatment requires that the entire surgical wound be radiated. The field size is much larger than the field size that would be provided with preoperative radiation. In addition to the larger field size, the poorly oxygenated postoperative field requires a higher dose of radiation than the well-oxygenated tumor before surgery. In contrast, the use of preoperative radiation is associated with lower total radiation dose and lower volume of tissue exposed to radiation (**Fig. 2**). The reason for the decreased field size is that the radiation can be contoured to the tumor itself, maximizing treatment of the viable peripheral cells that can implant in the wound, rather than treating the entire postoperative wound. Because the dose and field size are reduced, preoperative radiation may be associated with better functional outcomes and a lower fracture risk, especially if the periosteum is removed to obtain a negative surgical margin.

Disclosures: Paid consultant for Stryker and Corin.
Orthopaedic Oncology, University of Alabama at Birmingham Medical Center, Birmingham, AL, USA
E-mail address: hsiegel@uabmc.edu

Orthop Clin N Am 45 (2014) 99–107
http://dx.doi.org/10.1016/j.ocl.2013.08.006
0030-5898/14/$ – see front matter © 2014 Elsevier Inc. All rights reserved.

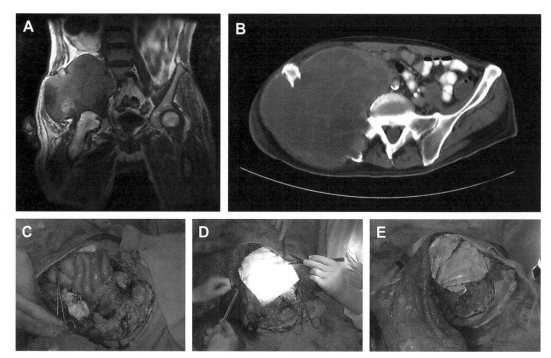

Fig. 1. (*A*) Coronal magnetic resonance imaging of the pelvis shows a massive telangiectatic osteosarcoma. The right hemipelvis is involved. The patient was treated with neoadjuvant chemotherapy followed by external hemipelvectomy. (*B*) CT scan showing a destructive lesion involving the right hemipelvis. No evidence of metastatic disease was noted on staging studies. (*C*) Intraoperative photo of resected right hemipelvis before abdominal wall reconstruction. Frozen section was performed at the margins of the mass and was negative for malignancy. (*D*) Soft tissue reconstruction was performed with a synthetic mesh graft. (*E*) The mesh graft was used to support the abdominal muscles and allows for neovascularization due to its porosity.

However, giving radiation before surgery is associated with a higher risk of wound-healing complications after surgery (**Fig. 3**).[3] Intensity modulated radiotherapy has the potential to reduce the surgical complication rate following preoperative radiation by protecting the superficial tissues that heal the wound as well as the underlying bone. However, intensity modulated radiotherapy requires a collaborative team of surgeons, radiation oncologists, and physicists to permit precise targeted radiotherapy delivery to very select volumes. This review covers the application of wound vacuum-assisted closure (VAC), silver-plated dressings, and hyperbaric oxygen treatment (HBOT) in the orthopedic oncology patient with a complex open wound.

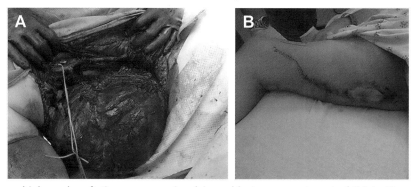

Fig. 2. (*A*) Large high-grade soft tissue sarcoma involving adductor compartment of thigh. The patient underwent preoperative radiation treatment. (*B*) Two-week postoperative picture showing sutures in place and a zone of skin necrosis. This wound required a debridement, wound VAC treatment, followed by delayed closure.

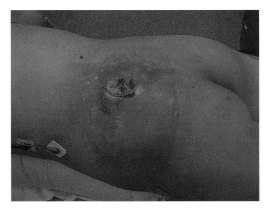

Fig. 3. Large synovial sarcoma involving sacro-iliac joint and L5 transverse process. A large zone of necrosis is seen with a fungating tumor. The patient had preoperative radiation with notable tumor size reduction.

RISK FACTORS FOR POOR WOUND HEALING

A problem wound is one that fails to progress normally through the typical stages of healing. It demonstrates poor granulation, persistent exudates, retarded or failure of/or failure of neo-epithelialization. Skin flaps and grafts fail to integrate with the underlying tissue, leading to retraction and death of the flap or graft and re-exposure of the original wound in its initial or a worsened state. In some cases, the overt cause of a problem wound is a surgical procedure in tissue that is intact but compromised. Multiple factors can contribute to the failure of a wound to heal. Low tissue oxygenation, caused either by decreased systemic oxygenation or by poor tissue perfusion, is foremost among these factors. Others include inflammation; infection; nutritional deficiencies; repetitive trauma; poor glucose and lipid control; hematologic, rheumatologic, and autoimmune disorders; use of certain medications; and social and economic concerns, such as alcohol and tobacco use, poverty, and homelessness. Therefore, treating any wound that is not healing properly must involve identification of all contributing factors and a focused attempt to eliminate or ameliorate each one.

Tobacco use bears special mention because it is common and avoidable. Tobacco contributes to the development of wounds, delays in healing, wound dehiscence, and infection. Nicotine causes vasoconstriction, resulting in local tissue hypoxia. Vasoconstriction in the microcirculation has been demonstrated within 5 to 10 minutes of smoking one cigarette, and microvascular flow is reduced by 30% to 38% after 2 cigarettes. Nicotine substitutes have the same effect. Smoking also appears to be correlated with long-term endothelial vasomotor alterations, endothelial dysfunction, accelerated atherosclerosis, platelet activation, and decrements in collagen synthesis, all of which contribute to poor wound healing in current and former smokers.[4]

WOUND VACUUM-ASSISTED CLOSURE TECHNOLOGY

As a negative margin is important to optimize local tumor control, resection of musculoskeletal tumors may result in large soft tissue defects that cannot be closed primarily and which may require prolonged dressing changes and complex surgical interventions for wound coverage.[5] Adequate wound debridement of necrotic tissue is essential, while preserving vital structures when possible. Soft tissue coverage may be performed at the same setting as the debridement or may be delayed after an interval period of wound VAC treatment (**Fig. 4**). The VAC is helpful to reduce soft tissue swelling and encourage the growth of vascularized granulation tissue. The disadvantages of wound VAC application include poor patient compliance because of discomfort, the need for frequent changes that may be uncomfortable, a foul smell, and difficulty with application in some anatomic areas. Although patient compliance has been improved with the development of mobile VAC units, areas such as the adductor compartment of the thigh and perineum remain a challenge.[6]

The wound VAC is generally applied to the surgical bed with the sponge in direct contact with muscle and/or fascia. An interposed synthetic covering is often helpful if neurovascular

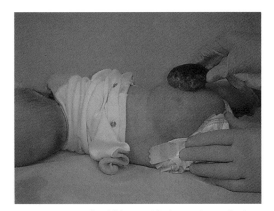

Fig. 4. A 6-month old boy with fungating soft tissue infantile fibrosarcoma. The mass shows discoloration and necrosis because of its rapid growth. The fungating portion appears to have outgrown its blood supply. A wide resection was performed followed by local soft tissue coverage and a wound VAC.

structures or bone are exposed in the wound. The author uses a petroleum gel–impregnated dressing to protect structures that may be compromised by direct sponge contact.[6] The skin surface may be coated with Mastisol or benzoin to help with dressing adherence. The sponge is contoured to fit the soft tissue defect without contact with the skin. In difficult areas such as the proximal adductor area, the sponge may be stapled to the skin at the periphery and stoma paste used under the sealant dressing for extra adherence.[6] The device is set to 125 mm Hg on continuous pressure; alternatively an intermittent pressure may be used.[7] The dressing is changed 3 times per week until the wound has healed enough for either a further surgical procedure such as skin grafting or soft tissue flap, or dressing changes alone.[6,7] Wounds with prior radiation exposure may reopen after initial closure and require long-term follow-up (**Fig. 5**).[6,7]

The author's group reported in 2007 that the hospital stay ($P<.025$), length of overall treatment ($P<.025$), number of operative debridements ($P<.05$), and success of wound closure without the need for soft tissue transposition ($P<.01$) were found to be significantly less in the wound VAC group compared with those not treated with the VAC device (**Fig. 6**).[6] The concern regarding the possible increased incidence of recurrence following soft tissue sarcoma resections is currently undergoing investigation. However, preliminary data have indicated that the VAC does not seem to be an impact on recurrence.

Bickels and colleagues[7] reviewed 23 patients with such defects treated with a vacuum-assisted wound closure system and compared the outcome of these patients with a control group. The study group included 15 women and 8 men who had their wounds located at the back (2), pelvic girdle (11), thigh (8), and leg (2). Treatment included sealed wound coverage with polyurethane foam and overlying tape connected to a vacuum pump. This system was disconnected and changed every 48 hours for 7 to 19 days, after which all defects were reduced in size by an average of 25% and covered with a viable granulation tissue. This viable granulation tissue allowed primary closure in 7 patients, primary closure with skin grafting in 14 patients, and healing by secondary intention in 2 patients. Compared with the control group, patients in the study group had shorter hospital stays and number of surgical interventions and greater rates of primary wound closure. The use of vacuum-assisted wound closure facilitates wound healing and primary wound closure in patients who have a large soft tissue defect after resection of a musculoskeletal tumor.[6,7]

As a supplement to skin grafting and soft tissue flaps, the wound VAC has demonstrated a significant benefit.[3,6,7] By removing fluid from the surgical bed, and applying pressure against the graft, the VAC has gained acceptance in plastic surgery, in orthopedic surgery, and by multiple disciplines of oncologic surgery.

SILVER TOPICAL DRESSINGS

Ionic silver at a concentration of 10^{-9} to 10^{-6} mol/L is bactericidal, fungicidal, virucidal, and protozoicidal (http://ewma.org/fileadmin/user_upload/EWMA/pdf/Position_Documents/2006/English_pos_doc_2006.pdf),[8–10] although more resistant micro-organisms, such as spores, cysts, and mycobacteria, are less inactivated or not inactivated at all.[11–14] This broad-spectrum activity is beneficial for its use as a topical application. Although silver has been used for many centuries and in wound management, its bactericidal mechanisms of action are still not fully understood. Silver has now assumed a prominent position in wound care and it is therefore appropriate to examine this agent in more detail.[15,16]

Mechanism of Silver Action

To be effective, silver must interact with and penetrate into the micro-organism to reach its target sites. It is thought that silver ions may compete with other cations for adsorption on the cell.[3] Bacterial cells usually possess 2 types of uptake system for heavy-metal ions: a nonspecific system, which transports many types of ions across the cell membrane and a substrate-specific system, which transports only one or select ions and may be switched on or off by the cell under particular

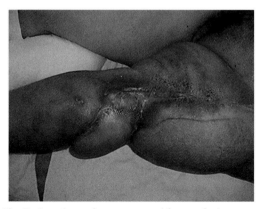

Fig. 5. A patient who was treated for a soft tissue sarcoma with wide resection, soft tissue flaps, and radiation. The patient began developing wound problems 10 years postoperatively. She was treated successfully with superficial debridement and a combination of silver negative pressure and the wound VAC.

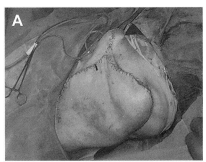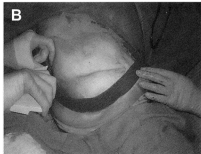

Fig. 6. (*A*) Intraoperative photo of closed hemipelvectomy. (*B*) An incision would VAC was applied to the incision. The drains were left in until there was minimal output. The wound healed without complication.

conditions.[4,17–19] Although not well documented for silver ions, it is possible that the bacterial cell cannot stop the transport of metal ions into the cytoplasm because nonspecific transporters cannot be switched off, which would explain the cytotoxicity of heavy metals against bacteria. The increased efficacy of silver sulfadiazine over silver nitrate may be explained by the apparent higher uptake of silver in the presence of a sulfonamide.[11,20,21] The molecular activity of silver is explained by its strong affinity for electron donor groups containing sulfur, oxygen, and nitrogen. This molecular activity of silver causes inhibition of bacterial enzymes and interferes with respiration at the cell membrane level.

The maximum level of available silver has been reported to be approximately 1 μg/mL in a physiologic environment in vitro.[22] Concentrations in excess of this are likely to serve only as a reserve against depletion in solution. Above this concentration, silver ions complex with anions, predominantly chloride, to form an insoluble inactive silver salt; there is no evidence that silver or silver salts are active in the dried state. The sustained efficacy of a formulation depends on the bioavailability of the silver ions and as such the delivery vehicle is of paramount importance to ensure a slow but sustained release of silver.

Most silver-containing dressings possess a high concentration of the agent.[23–26] The development of silver-containing dressings has in some cases allowed for the controlled delivery of silver, ensuring activity while controlling potential toxicity and side effects as the rate of silver release and deposition is controlled through hydration. One should note that dressings, including those containing silver, act as a barrier to wound contamination but they cannot eliminate micro-organisms already colonizing a wound.[27–29] The high level of silver reactivity might impair its penetration into the wound bed, which might be of concern if bacteria are residing in deeper tissue.

Microbiology of Silver

It is well recognized that silver nitrate shows strong activity against *Pseudomonas aeruginosa* but not necessarily as strongly against other micro-organisms.[9,13,20,28] From early work on silver nitrate compresses, Cason and colleagues[21] reported that silver nitrate failed to reduce colonization significantly with *Staphylococcus aureus* or coliform bacilli when compared with other antiseptic prophylaxis. There is relatively little information on the efficacy of silver and silver-containing products against anaerobes, although these organisms are present in chronic wounds. The combination of silver and a sulfonamide has been demonstrated to be synergistic against several bacteria commonly associated with burn infections.[10,11]

There is evidence for bacterial resistance to silver.[12] Therefore, exposure to silver might select resistant micro-organisms and this could play an important part in the predominance of intrinsically silver-resistant bacteria where silver is used widely. Jing and colleagues[8] reported the development of bacterial resistance to high concentrations of silver (>1024 ppm) by repeated exposures to increasing concentrations in vitro.

Use of Silver in Open Wounds

Advances in impregnation techniques and polymer technologies have fueled the latest interest in silver-based dressings and the application of silver-containing dressings in the management of chronic wounds is gaining momentum. There is a paucity of good-quality trials despite the extensive use of dressings worldwide. These modern products have developed from the understanding of the properties of silver and aim to improve conditions for wound healing primarily by controlling the wound bioburden. However, there are wide variations in the structure, formulation, and concentration of silver used in these products. Dressings and preparations containing silver have a better antimicrobial efficacy than do silver nitrate or silver sulfadiazine alone.

Cytotoxicity has been recognized with the use of silver cream and ointments.[9,15] In vitro keratinocyte toxicity has been described with silver-containing dressings in some studies but not others, indicating the choice of keratinocyte cell type and methodology is important.[9,15] In vivo studies and clinical evaluations of such silver dressings showed no tissue toxicity. The cytotoxicity of silver sulfadiazine is associated with a release of the sulfonamide rather than silver, and it has been associated with severe blood and skin disorders (burning, itching, and rashes).[20,22] Leucopenia and argyria (skin decolorization resulting from elemental silver deposition) have also been recognized.

In addition, using certain types of dressing, Aquacel Ag (Convatec, Princeton, NJ, USA), might enhance removal and inactivation of microorganisms by sequestration (retention) within the dressing matrix. The use of early silver formulations, such as solutions and creams, for treating open wounds was associated with several unwanted effects.

Silver plating technology is a novel application of silver to assist with wound healing. A recent study by the author's group evaluating the impact of a silver negative pressure dressing in conjunction with the wound VAC had a statistically significant impact on wound healing in massive wounds of the pelvis and extremities as compared with a similar cohort of patients treated with wound VAC alone (**Fig. 7**).[30] Specifically, hospitalization, the number of surgical procedures, and a reduction of discomfort with wound VAC changes were all found to be significantly impacted. The

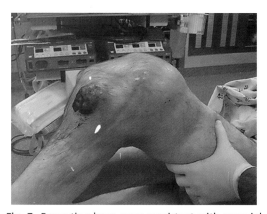

Fig. 7. Fungating knee mass consistent with synovial sarcoma. The patient underwent an above-knee amputation and healed without complication. A negative pressure silver dressing and wound VAC were used until complete wound healing at 10 days.

negative pressure silverlon dressing is placed in direct contact with the wound and overlaps the skin by 2 to 3 cm. The VAC sponge is placed on top of the silver dressing and contoured to the shape of the wound. Generally, 1 cm of silver negative pressure dressing extends past the area of the sponge. This silver negative pressure dressing protects the skin from maceration from the sponge. It appears that the silver negative pressure dressing inhibits a common foul smell from the wound VAC dressing and facilitates the dressing change by inhibiting granulation tissue penetration into the sponge. In the author's series, no black discoloration of the tissue was observed.[30] A study to evaluate the impact of a silver negative pressure and wound VAC on surgical incisions is currently ongoing at the author's institution. The preliminary results are highly promising in terms of infection reduction and reduction of hospital stay.

HBOT

HBOT has seen a resurgence of interest in recent years, with more medical centers building facilities and more physicians becoming board-certified in undersea and hyperbaric medicine. The reason for the growing interest is better understanding of the role of hypoxia in wound healing and an appreciation for the role of HBOT in reversing tissue hypoxia and enhancing the healing process, which has resulted in several new evidence-based indications for HBOT. Inspired by reports of successful treatment of gas gangrene and its potential in facilitating open-heart surgery and organ transplantation, several academic institutions constructed large hyperbaric research facilities in the mid-1960s.[31–34] As other means of accomplishing heart surgery and organ transplantation were developed, academic interest in hyperbaric medicine waned, although some commercial entities offered HBOT for off-label maladies including wrinkles, hair loss, and impotence. Thus, during the 1970s and 1980s, legitimate use of HBOT was limited to treatment of gas gangrene, decompression sickness, cerebral air embolism, and carbon monoxide poisoning.[35–37] Over the last 2 decades, however, there has been a resurgence of interest in HBOT.

The greatest impetus for growth in hyperbaric medicine practice has been better understanding of the role of hypoxia in nonhealing wounds and an appreciation for the role of HBOT in reversing tissue hypoxia and enhancing wound healing.[38] This impetus has resulted in several new evidence-based indications for HBOT, all of which share the therapeutic basis of correcting tissue hypoxia. The 2 medical conditions that are currently contributing most to the growing interest in hyperbaric medicine are chronic diabetic foot ulcers, tissue necrosis, osteomyelitis, amputations, and delayed radiation injury, which is associated with bone and soft tissue necrosis.[38,39]

Mechanism of Action

The dramatic increase in the arterial oxygen during HBOT creates a steep diffusion gradient favoring oxygen movement to tissue and increasing the diffusion distance of oxygen. At $3\times$ normal atmospheric pressure, for example, the diffusion distance from the precapillary arteriole into the extravascular compartment is increased from 64 μm to 240 μm. This increase is thought to enable a smaller number of capillaries to deliver oxygen to a larger volume of tissue.

HBOT promotes wound healing in several ways, including intermittent correction of tissue hypoxia and direct enhancement of fibroblast proliferation, collagen synthesis, neovascularization, and epithelialization.[38] It also reduces local tissue edema by causing vasoconstriction of both arterial and venous vessels. HBOT also improves the host immune response. It is toxic to anaerobes and promotes leukocyte bactericidal action against both gram-positive and gram-negative aerobes.[39] In addition, HBOT enhances the transport of aminoglycoside antibiotics across the bacterial cell wall, enhancing the efficacy of these drugs, which is inhibited in vivo by local tissue hypoxia.[10]

HBOT raises the low-tissue oxygen tensions in infected bone to normal or above-normal levels and stimulates osteoblast and osteoclast function, which is impaired under hypoxic conditions. It also up-regulates the gene expression for the platelet-derived growth factor β receptor, which may be one of the mechanisms by which HBOT enhances angiogenesis.

Hyperbaric Oxygen and Radiation Therapy

HBOT has been used successfully for 30 years to treat the complications of delayed radiation injury.[38,40] Delayed radiation injury is usually seen 6 months or more after radiation and is characterized by endarteritis, hypocellularity, and severe secondary fibrosis.

Wound healing in irradiated tissue is inhibited both by the hypoxia resulting from endarteritis and by the absence of cells essential for wound repair. HBOT stimulates angiogenesis in irradiated tissue, resulting in increased vascularity. Increased oxygen tensions in the irradiated tissue accompany this increased vascularity because patients progress through a series of hyperbaric treatments. In an animal model, the vascular density of even irradiated bone has been shown to increase with HBOT.[40] Increased cellular density also has been demonstrated in heavily irradiated tissue in humans.[37,38,40] The beneficial effect of HBOT on irradiated tissue is likely to involve all 3 mechanisms: stimulating angiogenesis, reducing fibrosis and increasing cellular density, and mobilizing stem cells.

HBOT and Surgery

Although spontaneous necrosis of soft tissue or bone in the irradiated field may occur, more often, complications of delayed radiation injury happen because of surgical procedures in the irradiated field. Based on the results of current research, a case may be made for preoperative HBOT to improve the outcome of any major surgical procedure that is to occur in a field that was heavily irradiated.[40]

Serious wound complications are common after head and neck surgeries within a previously irradiated field. In a series of patients for whom surgery was planned to repair radiation necrosis wounds or to resect recurrent cancer, a marked reduction was reported in the incidence of wound infection, wound dehiscence, and delayed healing when HBOT was used before and after surgery, compared with controls. However, patients requiring urgent salvage surgery for recurrent cancer in an irradiated field may not have the option of pretreatment. HBOT still has a role in reducing wound complications in these patients. When surgical resection is performed for laryngeal or pharyngeal cancers in previously irradiated fields, starting HBOT when it is evident that the wounds are not healing results in much improved outcomes compared with historical controls. An even greater reduction in complications is associated with starting HBOT immediately after surgery, without waiting for evidence of wound complications. More research is needed to identify the patients at greatest risk for and the procedures most associated with serious postoperative wound complications. Given the cost of a major flap procedure that fails (initial surgical costs, prolonged hospitalization, repeat debridements, and a second reconstructive procedure), for example, it is likely to be less expensive to undertake a coordinated plan of surgery and HBOT.

HBO can stimulate healing in refractory wounds and irradiated tissues. Therapy for refractory diabetic wounds is likely to reduce the risk of lower extremity amputation by 2 to 3 times, with an absolute rate of major amputation reductions of about 20% (eg, 11% vs 32%) and a number needed to treat of about 4.[38,39]

Other Indications for Use of HBOT

Hyperbaric medicine has grown over the past 2 decades primarily because of its efficacy for treating problem wounds. It has proved to be especially helpful for diabetic patients with chronic lower extremity wounds and for patients with cancer with healing problems caused by delayed radiation injury. Future potential orthopedic indications include periarticular soft tissue joint injury from multiple surgeries, trauma, and infection. HBOT will also likely have a role in the management of infections of the spine and pelvis.

HBOT is used on occasion to treat compromised flaps and grafts. At the author's institution, HBOT is commonly used for irradiated wounds in the treatment of sarcomas, particularly if they have undergone a prior unplanned excision. In this situation, often a wider resection is needed because of compromised or contaminated compartments and more adjuvant radiation may be needed to assist with local control than if resected initially with a negative surgical margin. Another growing indication is in the management of the patient with an infected total joint replacement. The implants are generally removed with an interval articulating spacer placed and during the course of antibiotic treatment, the patients are often referred for HBOT to assist with local tissue viability and antibiotic delivery.

SUMMARY

Using a multifactorial approach to the management of massive wounds will likely facilitate healing of massive, complex wounds as a result of tumor, trauma, and/or infection. The combination of HBOT, wound VAC therapy, and silver dressings has great potential and seems to reduce the morbidity and cost of wound management. Future randomized studies are needed to understand the impact of each modality better. Studying sarcoma patients and the complexity associated with wound care due to soft tissue loss, prior radiation exposure, and immunosuppression from chemotoxicity will likely lead to future improvements and the development of other modalities to improve wound care.

REFERENCES

1. Feldmeier JJ. Chapter 19: problem wounds: the irradiated wound. In: Sheffield PJ, Fife CE, Smith AP, editors. Wound care practice. Flagstaff (AZ): Best Publishing Company; 2004. p. 369–88.

2. Marx RE. Radiation injury to tissue. In: Kindwall EP, editor. Hyperbaric medicine practice. 2nd edition. Flagstaff (AZ): Best Publishing Company; 1999. p. 665–723.

3. Rosenberg LA, Esther RJ, Erfanian K, et al. Wound complications in preoperatively irradiated soft-tissue sarcomas of the extremities. Int J Radiat Oncol Biol Phys 2013;85(2):432–7.

4. Silverstein P. Smoking and wound healing. Am J Med 1992;93(1A):22S–4S.

5. Davidge KM, Wunder J, Tomlinson G, et al. Function and health status outcomes following soft tissue reconstruction for limb preservation in extremity soft tissue sarcoma. Ann Surg Oncol 2010;17(4):1052–62.

6. Siegel HJ, Long JL, Watson KM, et al. Vacuum assisted closure for radiation-associated complications. J Surg Oncol 2007;96(7):575–82.

7. Bickels J, Kollender Y, Wittig JC, et al. Vacuum-assisted wound closure after resection of musculoskeletal tumors. Clin Orthop Relat Res 2005;441:346–50.

8. Jing H, Yu Z, Li L. Antibacterial properties and corrosion resistance of Cu and Ag/Cu porous materials. J Biomed Mater Res A 2008;87(1):33–7.

9. Silver S. Bacterial silver resistance: molecular biology and uses and misuse of silver compounds. FEMS Microbiol Rev 2003;27:341–53.

10. Parsons D, Bowler PG, Myles V, et al. Silver antimicrobial dressings in wound management: a comparison of antibacterial, physical and chemical characteristics. Wounds 2005;17(8):222–32.

11. Richards ME, Taylor RG, Xing DK, et al. An evaluation of the antibacterial activities of combinations of sulphonamides, trimethoprim, dibromopropamidine, and silver nitrate compared with uptakes by selected bacteria. J Pharm Sci 1991;80(9):861–7.

12. Nies DH. Microbial heavy-metal resistance. Appl Microbiol Biotechnol 1999;51(6):730–50.

13. Russell AD, Hugo WB. Antimicrobial activity and action of silver. Prog Med Chem 1994;31:351–71.

14. Sibbald RG, Browne AC, Coutts P, et al. Screening evaluation of an ionized nanocrystalline silver in chronic wound care. Ostomy Wound Manage 2001;47(10):38–43.

15. Lansdown AB, Williams A. How safe is silver in wound care? J Wound Care 2004;13(4):131–6.

16. Lansdown AB, Sampson B, Laupattarakasem P, et al. Silver aids healing in the sterile skin wound: experimental studies in the laboratory rat. Br J Dermatol 1997;137(5):728–35.

17. Liau SY, Read DC, Pugh WJ, et al. Interaction of silver nitrate with readily identifiable groups: relationship to the antibacterial action of silver. Lett Appl Microbiol 1997;25:279–83.

18. Richards RM. Antimicrobial action of silver nitrate. Microbios 1981;31:83–91.

19. Percival SL, Bowler PG, Russell D, et al. Bacterial resistance to silver in wound care. J Hosp Infect 2005;60(1):1–7.

20. Coward JE, Carr HS, Rosenkranz HS. Silver sulphadiazine: effect on the growth and ultrastructure of Staphylococci. Chemotherapy 1973;19:348–53.

21. Cason JS, Jackson DM, Lowbury EJ, et al. Antiseptic and aseptic prophylaxis for burns: use of silver nitrate and of isolators. BMJ 1966;2:1288–94.

22. Lam PK, Chan ES, Ho WS, et al. In vitro cytotoxicity testing of a nanocrystalline silver dressing (Acticoat) on cultured keratinocytes. Br J Biomed Sci 2004; 61(3):125–7.

23. Dunn K, Edwards-Jones V. The role of Acticoat with nanocrystalline silver in the management of burns. Burns 2004;30(Suppl 1):S1–9.

24. Walker M, Cochrane CA, Bowler PG. Silver deposition and tissue staining associated with wound dressings containing silver. Ostomy Wound Manage 2006;52(1):42–50.

25. Jones S, Bowler PG, Walker M. Antimicrobial activity of silver-containing dressing is influenced by dressing conformability with wound surface. Wounds 2005;17(9):263–70.

26. Burrell RE. A scientific perspective on the use of topical silver preparations. Ostomy Wound Manage 2003;49(Suppl 5A):19–24.

27. Jones SA, Bowler PG, Walker M, et al. Controlling wound bioburden with a novel silver-containing Hydrofiber dressing. Wound Repair Regen 2004; 12(3):288–94.

28. Wright JB, Lam K, Hansen D, et al. Efficacy of topical silver against burn wound pathogens. Am J Infect Control 1999;27:344–50.

29. Malliard JY, Hartmann P. Silver as an antimicrobial: facts and gaps in knowledge. Crit Rev Microbiol 2012. [Epub ahead of print].

30. Siegel HJ, Herrera D, Gay J. Massive wounds of the pelvis and extremities managed by a silver negative pressure dressing and wound VAC. Clin Orthop Relat Res, in press.

31. Thom SR. Hyperbaric oxygen therapy. J Intensive Care Med 1989;4:58–74.

32. Valko M, Leibfritz D, Moncol J, et al. Free radicals and antioxidants in normal physiological functions and human disease. Int J Biochem Cell Biol 2007;39:44–84.

33. Dennog C, Radermacher P, Barnett YA, et al. Antioxidant status in humans after exposure to hyperbaric oxygen. Mutat Res 1999;428:83–9.

34. Dennog C, Hartmann A, Frey G, et al. Detection of DNA damage after hyperbaric oxygen (HBO) therapy. Mutagenesis 1996;11:605–9.

35. Mathieu D. Handbook on hyperbaric medicine. Dordrecht (The Netherlands): Springer; 2006.

36. Neuman TS, Thom SR. Physiology and medicine of hyperbaric oxygen therapy. Philadelphia: Saunders-Elsevier; 2008.

37. Gesell LB. Hyperbaric oxygen therapy indications. 12th edition. Durham (NC): Undersea and Hyperbaric Medical Society; 2008.

38. Goldman RJ. Hyperbaric oxygen therapy for wound healing and limb salvage: a systematic review. PM R 2009;1:471–89.

39. Doctor N, Pandya S, Supe A. Hyperbaric oxygen therapy in diabetic foot. J Postgrad Med 1991;38:112–4.

40. Marx RE, Ehler WJ, Tayapongsak P, et al. Relationship of oxygen dose to angiogenesis induction in irradiated tissue. Am J Surg 1990;160:519–24.

The Practicing Orthopedic Surgeon's Guide to Managing Long Bone Metastases

Felix H. Cheung, MD

KEYWORDS

- Long bone metastasis • Skeletally related events • Pathologic fracture • Evaluation and treatment
- Practical primer • Bone tumor

KEY POINTS

- A thorough evaluation should be conducted to confirm metastatic disease before definitive fixation.
- Placement of the biopsy is crucial to prevent further morbidity.
- Prophylactic fixation (long nails) for impending fractures is preferred.
- Cemented arthroplasty options for periarticular pathologic fractures and long nails for other kinds of fractures including peritrochanteric are preferred.

INTRODUCTION

Treatment of skeletal metastases is a significant part of cancer care in the United States. The estimated prevalence of metastatic bone disease in the United States is at least 280,000 per year and is expected to increase as medical management improves overall survivorship.[1] Postmortem analysis shows that around 70% of all patients with breast and prostate cancer have skeletal metastases, and it involves between 35% and 42% of patients with lung, thyroid, and renal cancer.[2] The economic costs of treatment of metastatic bone disease in the United States per year are an estimated $12.6 billion, which is 17% of the total annual cost of cancer treatments.[3]

The purpose of this article is to review the presentation, workup, and treatment options for metastatic disease to the long bones. Seven scenarios are presented to help the practicing orthopedist identify and treat metabolic bone disease safely.

PRESENTATION

The typical patient will present with a history of a primary carcinoma and bony pain. Occasionally (about 15% of the time), the patient will present with no known primary. The bone pain is typically described as a "gnawing, tooth-achy" pain, or "night" pain. Pain with weight-bearing or sharp pain is concerning for impending pathologic fracture. The most common locations for metastatic disease include the spine, pelvic girdle, shoulder girdle, and distal femur.[2] Metastasis distal to the knee and elbow is rare except for lung cancer.[4]

A thorough history and physical examination are mandatory, including past medical history, smoking history, exposure to carcinogens and radiation, and a full review of symptoms including constitutional symptoms (**Table 1**).

Physical examination should include an examination of the limb, looking for causes of pain other than cancer, as well as goiter examination, lymph node examination, auscultation of the lungs, breast examination, and digital rectal examination (**Table 2**).

LABORATORY WORKUP

Standard laboratory workup for patients without a known primary include CBC with Diff, CMP, U/A, ESR/CRP, PSA, SPEP/UPEP, PTH (**Table 3**).[5]

Department of Orthopaedic Surgery, Joan C Edwards School of Medicine, Marshall University, 1600 Medical Center Dr, Ste G500, Huntington, WV 25701, USA
E-mail address: cheungf@marshall.edu

Orthop Clin N Am 45 (2014) 109–119
http://dx.doi.org/10.1016/j.ocl.2013.09.003
0030-5898/14/$ – see front matter © 2014 Elsevier Inc. All rights reserved.

Table 1
Review of systems

Review of System	Possible Malignancy
Fevers, sweats, chills, weight loss	Lymphoma
Shortness of breath, pleuritic pain, hemoptysis	Lung
Voiding difficulty	Prostate
Hematuria	Renal
Breast discharge or mass	Breast
Rectal bleeding, anemia	Colon

Table 2
Physical examination

Physical Examination	Possible Malignancy
Jaundice	Liver
Neck nodules	Thyroid
Axillary nodules, breast lump, or discharge	Breast
Dull auscultation of the lungs	Lung
Splenomegaly	Lymphoma
Positive digital rectal examination	Prostate

Table 3
Laboratory orders

Lab	Possible Malignancy
CBC with Diff	Multiple myeloma, leukemias
CMP: Ca/Alk Phos	Amount of bony involvement, prognosis
U/A	Renal from hematuria
ESR/CRP	Inflammation from infection, tumor burden
PSA	Prostate
SPEP/UPEP	Multiple myeloma
PTH	Metabolic bone disease

Abbreviations: CBC, Complete Blood Count with differential; CMP, Comprehensive metabolic panel; ESR/CRP, sedimentation rate/C-Reactive Protein; PTH, Parathyroid hormone; SPEP/UPEP, Serum Protein Electrophoresis/Urine Protein Electrophoresis; U/A, urinalysis.

IMAGING WORKUP

Good radiographs, focused on the tumor in orthogonal planes, are required for proper assessment of the lesion. Axial imaging (computed tomography [CT] or magnetic resonance imaging scan) can be helpful in determining the amount of bony destruction, extent of the tumor, risk of fracture, and choice of implant. A whole body bone scan is useful for determining other sites of metastatic disease. If multiple myeloma is known or suspected, a skeletal survey is needed[6] because many of the lesions will not be osteoblastic.

If the primary is unknown, radiographs, CT scan of the chest, abdomen, and pelvis, and a whole body bone scan are recommended. Approximately 85% of primary tumors can be identified in this manner.[7] Mammography for women and thyroid ultrasound can be helpful if the physical examination findings are supportive (**Table 4**).

PATHOLOGIC WORKUP

A biopsy is recommended if the primary is unknown, or if it is a solitary lesion. This biopsy is to ensure that the tumor is not a primary bone sarcoma or that there is not a secondary primary. The biopsy can be performed using a core needle technique (with or without interventional radiology)

Table 4
Imaging orders

Imaging	Use
X-rays	Screening, surgical planning
CT or magnetic resonance imaging of bone	Risk of fracture, extent of disease, choice of implant
Whole body bone scan	Screen for other sites of bony metastatic disease
Skeletal survey	Screen for multiple myeloma
CT chest/abdomen/pelvis	Look for solid organ primary carcinoma
Mammography	Screen for breast cancer primary (if examination is suspicious)
Thyroid ultrasound	Screen for thyroid cancer primary (if examination is suspicious)

Table 5 Biopsy options		
Biopsy Type	Advantages	Disadvantages
Open (1–3 cm incision)	Most tissue, most accurate	Most contamination from size of incision
Core needle (10–14 g)	Maintains architecture of tissue Little contamination	Less accurate due to less tissue (80%)
Fine needle aspirate (24 g)	Little contamination	Least accurate due to loss of architecture of tissue

or an open procedure (**Table 5**). If surgical fixation is already planned, then a separate, well-planned open biopsy with frozen section immediately before the fixation should be considered. The case should not proceed until the pathology report is returned, confirming metastatic disease. If the frozen pathology specimen is inconclusive, then the case should be aborted until the final pathology report is returned.

Reamings

Q: Is sending the reamings from the nailing ok for the biopsy?

A: Sending reamings is not recommended for 2 reasons. First, the quality of the tissue has been compromised by the destructive shearing forces of the reamer, leading to a less accurate result. Second, the entire femur is now contaminated by tumor, which may complicate reconstructive options if the tumor was not a carcinoma. A separate open biopsy and waiting for the results before taking the steps for fixation (incision extension, reaming) are recommended.

It is recommended that the biopsy be performed at institutions that have the capability to treat the definitive disease because a poorly placed biopsy can significantly affect the morbidity of subsequent procedures,[8] affecting the amount of soft tissue and bony resection, function after surgery, and recurrence. Poorly placed CT-guided needle biopsies can also contaminate tissue planes, necessitating a change in the subsequent surgery and morbidity.

Treatments can vary substantially based on the histology. Some primary tumor-specific information is provided in **Table 6**.

How to do a biopsy

Q: What are the keys to a well-placed biopsy?

A:

1 Place the biopsy tract in-line with the planned incision line from the definitive surgery

2 Use longitudinal incisions (incisions parallel to the underlying compartment)

3 Go through soft tissue compartments, not around them, to contaminate less tissue

4 Undermine as little tissue as possible

5 Get meticulous hemostasis, or place a drain to prevent hematoma and spread of tumor

6 Get a frozen section to confirm pathologic tissue on the specimen

TREATMENTS

Treatments for bony metastasis depend on the clinical presentation and tumor type. If the patient is asymptomatic, then observation with repeat radiographs in 3 to 4 months may be all that is needed. Use of a bisphosphonate or a RANK L inhibitor should be considered to reduce skeletally related events or fractures.[10] If the patient is symptomatic, but there is no risk for pathologic fracture, then radiation therapy may be helpful for palliation of the symptoms.[11] Patients with multiple lesions may be candidates for radiopharmaceutical treatments.[12]

Surgical management of the metastatic disease centers on preventing fractures or encouraging

ASTRO Guidelines

ASTRO Guidelines for Palliative Skeletal Metastasis[11]

30 Gy in 10 fractions OR 8 Gy in 1 fraction

Table 6
Primary tumor-specific information

	Radiosensitive?	Chemosensitive?	Hormone Sensitive	Bloody?	Fracture Heal Rate[9]	Metastatectomy?
Breast	Yes	Yes	Yes	No	37%	No
Kidney	Only at higher doses	Yes	No	Yes, embolize before open procedures	44%	Yes
Lung	Yes	Yes	No	No	0	No
Prostate	Yes	Yes	Yes	No	?	No
Thyroid	Yes, use radioiodine therapy	Yes	No	Yes, embolize before open procedures	?	Yes
Multiple myeloma	Yes	Yes	No	Possibly, consider embolize before open procedures	67%	No

Table 7
Mirels criteria

	1	2	3
Location	Upper extremities	Lower extremities	Peritrochanteric
Size	<1/3 cortex	>1/3, but <2/3 cortex	>2/3 cortex
Pain	Mild	Moderate	Severe or functional
Matrix	Blastic	Mixed	Lytic

healing after fractures. Treating impending fractures before they break is associated with less blood loss, shorter hospital stay, better function, and longer survival, although these were retrospective studies,[13,14] This treatment can be accomplished with prophylactic fixation using intramedullary (IM) nails, or periarticular plates. Occasionally the entire portion of the bone may need to be removed and replaced with a cemented endoprothesis.

The decision of whether a lesion requires prophylactic fixation can be performed in a methodical fashion. The most commonly used criteria is Mirels criteria (**Table 7**).[15]

Each row is assigned a score of 1 to 3. The rows are added up, and if the score is less than 8, there is a less than 15% chance of fracture and no prophylactic fixation is needed. If the score is greater than 8, there is a greater than 30% chance of fracture, and prophylactic fixation is recommended. If the score is equal to 8, there is no recommendation. These criteria have been externally validated.[16]

Some centers are using a CT-based structural rigidity analysis to quantify the weakness of a bone compared with the other side. Early results show better sensitivity and specificity compared with Mirels criteria.[17]

The decision for surgery and the kind of fixation can be distilled into 4 key thought processes, as illustrated in **Table 8**.

Whether the patient will survive the surgical procedure is based on the patient's preoperative health. One common assessment of preoperative health is the Goldman classification[18] to give a risk for perioperative major cardiac complications. This classification is based on cardiac, respiratory, and other medical factors and is often performed by the anesthesiologist or the medical consultant. An estimation of the life expectancy for the patient with pathologic fractures is difficult to determine. The most accurate predictors (in order) were clinician estimation, hemoglobin, number of visceral metastasis, and Eastern Cooperative Oncology Group score, but overall it was still only 18% accurate.[19]

Immediate functionality of the construct is important because the patient's lifespan may be limited. Therefore, constructs that rely on allograft healing,

bone healing, ingrowth into stems and cups, and so on are discouraged in favor of cemented constructs. Cementing must be done carefully, with low-viscosity cement, minimal pressurization, clean canals, and adequate patient hydration to reduce the rate of fat emboli.[20]

Classic teaching recommends prophylactic management of the entire bone if it can be done without undue difficulty. Two recent retrospective articles have questioned this teaching. Alvi and Damron[21] looked at 96 long bone metastases treated with long intramedullary nails or long cemented stems. Only 1/96 (1.04%) developed new metastasis distal to the original lesion, whereas there was a 12.5% rate of physiologic complications from using a longer implant that may have been avoided with a shorter implant. Most of these complications were attributed to cementing long-stemmed prostheses.

Table 8
Decisions for surgery

Will the patient survive and will the recovery time be less than the expected life expectancy?	Y: Consider surgery N: Consider nonoperative management
Will the surgical construct allow immediate functionality?	Y: Consider that construct N: Consider something else if reasonable
Will the surgical construct be prophylactic against future metastatic disease in the same bone?	Y: Consider that construct N: Consider something else if reasonable
Will the surgical construct allow for postoperative palliative radiation for the entire operative field?	Y: Consider that construct N: Consider something else if reasonable

Xing and coworkers[22] retrospectively looked at 206 lesions in the proximal femur treated with cemented arthroplasty with varying length stems. Five of 206 femurs demonstrated new distal lesions (2.4%), but there was a significant difference in the complication rates of the long-stemmed prosthesis compared with the shorter ones (28% vs 16%). Consensus of most surgeons is to use a long IM nail if it is indicated. If cemented arthroplasty is chosen, standard length stems should be considered because using long-stemmed, cemented prostheses may cause more complications than prevent early failure.

The use of radiation after surgery is helpful to prevent recurrence. Townsend and colleagues[23] have shown a reduction from 15% to 3% of local recurrence after radiation. Because radiation can retard the rate of bone healing and bony ingrowth into prostheses, it is recommended that the surgical construct not rely on bony growth for immediate return to function. It is also recommended that the radiation field cover the entire operative field, including the entire intramedullary nail if applicable.[24] There is surprisingly a lack of good published data indicating whether this reduces local recurrence.

Consideration for performing an open curettage of the tumor before fixation should be made. Advantages include debulking of the tumor, allowing for better radiotherapy response, and the ability to use bone cement to augment the fixation, allowing for earlier return to function. Disadvantages include longer surgical time with more blood loss, increasing the surgical risk to the patient. There are no conclusive data to support or reject either course of action.

POSTOPERATIVE MANAGEMENT

Standard orthopedic postoperative care is expected. Medical management consultation may be useful to manage the higher level of medical complexity of these patients. Proper pain management and deep vein thrombosis prophylaxis is important. At least 24 hours of postoperative antibiotics is needed. There are currently no good published data demonstrating a change in infection rates if antibiotics are extended beyond that time. Early weight-bearing if possible is encouraged. If the patient has received chemotherapy or radiation to the affected wound, an incisional wound vacuum dressing and leaving the sutures in longer than normal to accommodate the slower healing rates may be helpful.

Scenario 1: Painful Bone Lesion in <40 year old

A 36-year-old woman presents to the clinic with a painful right knee. She has no history of cancer.

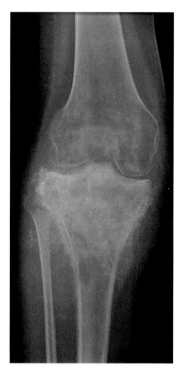

Fig. 1. This patient was ultimately biopsied and discovered to have Ewing sarcoma.

Radiographs (**Fig. 1**) demonstrate a lesion in the proximal tibia.

Our recommendation is to refer to an orthopedic oncologist, as this may represent primary bone cancer.

NCCN guidelines
NCCN 2013 Guidelines
Age <40 with a bone lesion = refer to orthopedic oncologist

Scenario 2: Painful Bone Lesion in >40 Year Old

A 41-year-old woman presents to the clinic with a painful left shoulder. She has no history of cancer. Radiographs (**Fig. 2**) demonstrate a lesion in the proximal humerus.

Our recommendation is to evaluate for metastatic disease, including laboratory tests (CBC w/diff, CMP, ESR, CRP, SPEP, UPEP, PSA if male patient) and additional imaging (CT chest/Abd/pelvis; whole body bone scan; mammography, if female patient) and a biopsy of the lesion if a primary carcinoma is suspected. Referral to an orthopedic oncologist is recommended if no primary is found.

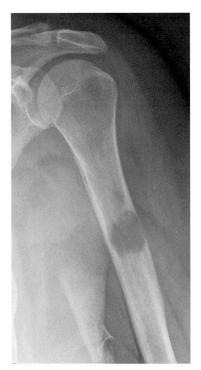

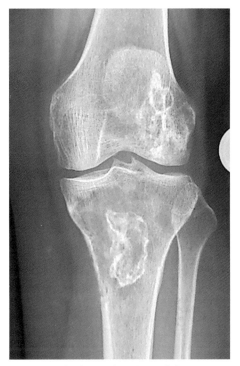

Fig. 2. This patient was discovered to have liver masses on CT scan. Biopsy ultimately showed hepatocellular carcinoma.

Fig. 3. Patient had no other sites of disease on staging. Biopsy revealed high-grade sarcoma of bone, NOS.

Scenario 3: New Painful Bone Lesion with Remote History of Cancer

A 50-year-old woman presents with a painful right proximal tibia. She has a history of non-Hodgkin lymphoma and has been in remission for 20 years. Radiographs (**Fig. 3**) reveal a bony infarct, with a lytic lesion in the proximal tibia.

Our recommendation is to evaluate the patient as if this might represent a second primary and follow the recommendations in Scenario 2. The error is to assume it is the original primary without verifying with a workup or biopsy.

Scenario 4: Bone Lesion with Current/Recent History of Cancer

A 67-year-old woman with a recent history of breast cancer presents with a blastic lesion in the right hip (**Fig. 4**). It does not represent impending pathologic fracture according to Mirels criteria.

We recommend biopsy of a solitary metastasis for staging purposes, usually a CT-guided core needle biopsy to minimize morbidity. If there are multiple sites of metastasis, biopsy may be unnecessary. Once confirmed, we recommend radiation therapy if the lesions are painful, and

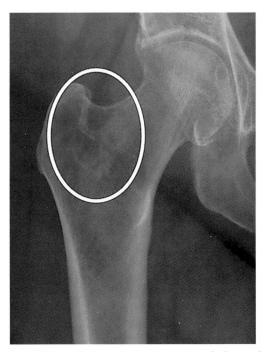

Fig. 4. This patient was asymptomatic and observed with serial radiographs. She received zolendronic acid for prevention of fracture.

observation in 3 to 4 months with radiographs if they are asymptomatic. The patient should receive a bisphosphonate or RANK L inhibitor either way.

Scenario 5: Bone Lesion with Impending Pathologic Fracture

A 52-year-old man with a recent diagnosis of multiple myeloma presents with severe hip pain with weight-bearing. Radiographs show a lytic, large lesion in the intertrochanteric region of the femur (**Fig. 5**). A skeletal survey shows multiple sites of disease.

Our assessment is that this is an impending pathologic fracture according to Mirels criteria. We recommend curettage and cement packing (if the patient can tolerate the longer surgery), prophylactic fixation spanning the entire hip and femur, and postoperative radiation after the wounds have healed.

Table 9 lists our preferences for treating each long bone with an impending pathologic fracture. For impending fractures, we prefer to preserve the soft tissue attachments to the bone and the articular cartilage for better function and lower infection rates, using bone cement and internal fixation as opposed to primary bone and joint replacement.

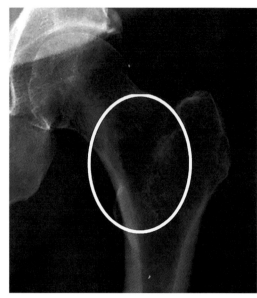

Fig. 5. This patient received a long cephalomedullary device for prevention of fracture.

Scenario 6: Bone Lesion with Pathologic Fracture

A 56-year-old woman presents to the clinic with a fracture through a lesion in the proximal humerus (**Fig. 6**). She has no history of cancer.

Table 9
Preferred treatments for impending pathologic fractures by location

		Impending Path Fracture
Long Bone	**Location**	**Treatment**
Humerus	Proximal	Proximal humeral plate or long proximal humeral nail
	Diaphyseal	IM nail
	Distal	Distal humeral plate
Radius	Proximal	Small fragment T plate or radial head arthroplasty
	Diaphyseal	Small fragment plate or flexible nail
	Distal	Distal radius plate
Ulna	Proximal	Olecranon plate
	Diaphyseal	Small fragment plate or flexible nail
	Distal	Small fragment plate
Femur	Proximal	Long cephalomedullary nail or cemented hemiarthroplasty
	Diaphyseal	Long cephalomedullary nail
	Distal	Distal femoral plate or long retrograde supracondylar nail
Tibia	Proximal	Proximal tibia plate
	Diaphyseal	IM nail
	Distal	Distal tibia plate
Fibula	Proximal	Nonsurgical
	Diaphyseal	Nonsurgical
	Distal	Distal fibula plate or retrograde screw

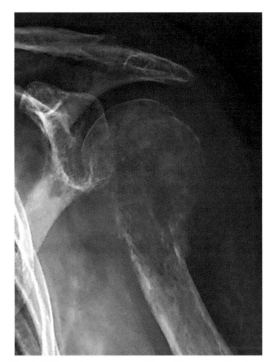

Fig. 6. This patient was considered for a proximal humerus replacement for her pathologic fracture, but declined due to health reasons.

We recommend that the appropriate staging as stated in Scenario 2 should be done, followed by a core needle biopsy done before surgery. Otherwise, if a biopsy is performed at the time of surgery and the pathology report is inconclusive or suggestive of sarcoma, we recommend halting the planned fixation and proceeding with nonoperative management until the final pathology report comes back.

Table 10 lists preferences for treating each long bone with a pathologic fracture. We tend to be more aggressive with endoprothesis use after a fracture has occurred due to the slow healing rates of pathologic fractures (see **Table 6**). All endoprotheses should be cemented.

Scenario 7: Time Distant Metastasis in Renal and Thyroid Cancer

An 86-year-old man with a history of renal cancer treated 7 years ago presents with a painful bony lesion in the distal femur (**Fig. 7**). Staging reveals no other sites of disease. Biopsy reveals renal cancer.

Our recommendation is to perform a metastatectomy with reconstruction. Metastatectomy for patients with renal or thyroid cancer who present with distant metastases greater than 5 years out demonstrate improved overall survivorship and there is

Table 10
Preferred treatments for pathologic fractures by location

Long Bone	Location	Treatment
		Pathologic Fracture
Humerus	Proximal	Proximal humerus replacement or proximal humeral plate with cement
	Diaphyseal	IM nail with cement
	Distal	Total elbow arthroplasty or distal humeral plate with cement
Radius	Proximal	Small fragment T plate with cement or proximal radial replacement
	Diaphyseal	Small fragment plate or flexible nail, with cement
	Distal	Distal radius plate with cement, or wrist fusion to ulna
Ulna	Proximal	Olecranon plate with cement or total elbow arthroplasty
	Diaphyseal	Small fragment plate or flexible nail, with cement
	Distal	Small fragment plate with cement or resection
Femur	Proximal	Head or neck: proximal femoral replacement, or calcar replacing hip replacement; Peritrochanteric: long cephalomedullary nail, with cement or proximal femur replacement
	Diaphyseal	Long cephalomedullary nail, with cement
	Distal	Distal femoral replacement, distal femoral plate with cement
Tibia	Proximal	Proximal tibia plate with cement, proximal tibial replacement
	Diaphyseal	IM nail with cement
	Distal	Distal tibia plate, amputation
Fibula	Proximal	Nonsurgical
	Diaphyseal	Nonsurgical
	Distal	Distal fibula plate or ankle fusion

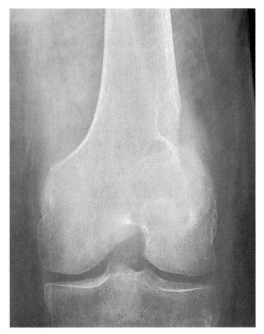

Fig. 7. This patient underwent a resection and distal femoral replacement.

growing evidence that it improves survivorship even if the timeframe is shorter than 5 years.[25,26]

SUMMARY

Skeletal metastases are relatively common and can be treated successfully by the practicing orthopedist. Key scenarios summarizing the most common situations are presented (also see **Table 11**) to help the surgeon care for his or her patient.

REFERENCES

1. Shuling Li, Peng Y, Weinhandl ED, et al. Estimated number of prevalent cases of metastatic bone disease in the US adult population. Clin Epidemiol 2012;4:87–93.
2. Coleman RE. Clinical features of metastatic bone disease and risk of skeletal morbidity. Clin Cancer Res 2006;12:6243s–9s.
3. Schulman KL, Kohles J. Economic burden of metastatic bone disease in the US. Cancer 2007;109:2334–42.
4. Healey JH, Turnbull AD, Miedema B, et al. Acrometastases: a study of twenty nine with osseous involvement of the hands and feet. J Bone Joint Surg Am 1986;16:743–6.
5. Jacofsky DJ, Frassica DA, Frassica FJ. Metastatic disease to bone. Hosp Physician 2004;39:21–8.
6. Ludwig H, Kumpan W, Sinzinger H. Radiography and bone scintigraphy in multiple myeloma; a comparative analysis. Br J Radiol 1982;55:173–81.
7. Rougraff BT, Kneisl JS, Simon MA. Skeletal metastasis of unknown origin. A prospective study of a diagnostic strategy. J Bone Joint Surg Am 1993;75(9):1276–81.
8. Mankin HJ, Mankin CJ, Simon MA. The hazards of the biopsy, revisited. Members of the Musculoskeletal Tumor Society. J Bone Joint Surg Am 1996;78(5):656–63.
9. Gainor BJ, Buchart P. Fracture healing in metastatic bone disease. Clin Orthop Relat Res 1983;178:297–302.
10. Ross JR, Saunders Y, Edmonds PM, et al. Systemic review of the role of bisphosphonates on skeletal morbidity in metastatic cancer. BMJ 2003;7413(327):469.
11. Lutz ST, Berk L, Chang E, et al. Palliative radiotherapy for bone metastases: an ASTRO evidence-based guideline. Int J Radiat Oncol Biol Phys 2011;79(4):965–76.
12. Petersen LJ, Lund L, Jonier M. Samarium-153 treatment of bone pain in patients with metastatic prostate cancer. Dan Med Bull 2010;57(6):A4154.
13. Ward WG, Holsenbeck S, Dorey FJ, et al. Metastatic disease of the femur: surgical treatment. Clin Orthop Relat Res 2003;(Suppl 415):S230–44.

Table 11
Key scenarios and treatments

Scenario	Situation	Treatment
1	<40 bone lesion	Refer to Ortho Onc
2	>40 new painful bone lesion	CT CAP, WBBS, laboratory tests, biopsy
3	New bone lesion, remote CA history	Treat like scenario 2
4	New bone lesion, current CA history	Biopsy, observe, radiate?, bisphos
5	New bone lesion, impending fracture	Biopsy, proph if not sarcoma
6	Pathologic fracture	Biopsy, replace or fix if not sarcoma
7	New time-distant metastasis for renal or thyroid	Consider metastatecomy

Abbreviations: Biopsy, Bisphosphonates; CAP, Chest/Abdomen/Pelvis; ortho Onc, Orthopaedic Oncologist; proph, Prophyllaxis; WBBS, Whole Body Bone Scan.

14. Katzer A, Meenen NM, Rueger JM. Surgery of skeletal metastases. Arch Orthop Trauma Surg 2002; 122(5):251–8.

15. Mirels H. Metastatic disease in long bones: a proposed scoring system for diagnosing impending pathologic fractures. Clin Orthop Relat Res 1989;249:256–64.

16. Damron TA, Morgan H, Prakash D, et al. Critical evaluation of Mirels' rating system for impending pathologic fractures. Clin Orthop Relat Res 2003;(Suppl 415):S201–7.

17. Snyder BD, Hauser-Kara DA, Hipp JA, et al. Predicting fracture through benign skeletal lesions with quantitative computed tomography. J Bone Joint Surg Am 2006;88:55–70.

18. Goldman L, Caldera DL, Nussbaum SR, et al. Multifactorial index of cardiac risk in noncardiac surgical procedures. N Engl J Med 1977;297:845.

19. Nathan SS, Healey JH, Mellano D, et al. Survival in patients operated on for pathologic fracture: implications for end-of-life orthopedic care. J Clin Oncol 2005;23(25):6072–82.

20. Randall RL, Aoki SK, Olson PR, et al. Complications of cemented long-stem hip arthroplasties in metastatic bone disease. Clin Orthop Relat Res 2006; 443:287–95.

21. Alvi HM, Damron TA. Prophylactic stabilization for bone metastases, myeloma, or lymphoma: do we need to protect the entire bone? Clin Orthop Relat Res 2013;471(3):706–14.

22. Xing Z, Moon BS, Satcher RL, et al. A long femoral stem is not always required in hip arthroplasty for patients with proximal femur metastases. Clin Orthop Relat Res 2013;471:1622–7.

23. Townsend PW, Rosenthal HG, Smalley SR, et al. Impact of postoperative radiation therapy and other perioperative factors on outcome after orthopaedic stabilization of impending or pathologic fractures due to metastatic disease. J Clin Oncol 1994;12: 2345–50.

24. The management of metastatic bone disease in the United Kingdom. Guidelines, British Association of Surgical Oncology. Eur J Surg Oncol 1999;25:2–23.

25. Ljungberg B. The role of metastasectomy in renal cell carcinoma in the era of targeted therapy. Curr Urol Rep 2013;14(1):19–25.

26. Pak H, Gourgiotis L, Chang WI, et al. Role of metastasectomy in the management of thyroid carcinoma: the NIH experience. J Surg Oncol 2003; 82(1):10–8.

Upper Extremity

Preface
Upper Extremity

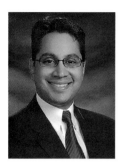

Asif M. Ilyas, MD
Editor

In this issue of the *Orthopedic Clinics of North America*, we present several interesting articles in the Upper Extremity section reviewing common shoulder and wrist pathologies:

McCormick et al present a detailed review of type II superior labral anterior to posterior tears and their arthroscopic management. A review of the pathology and comparative review of performing a biceps repair versus tenodesis is presented. Particular emphasis is placed on the challenge of treating this injury in overhead athletes.

Caggiano and Matullo have provided a comprehensive review of carpal instability of the wrist. They review the mechanism of injury of intercarpal ligaments, its diagnosis, and subsequent management with particular emphasis on recent evidence.

Cross and Matullo review Kienböck disease, also known as avascular necrosis or osteomalacia of the lunate. They identify the various advances in etiology, pathophysiology, and treatment for this insidious and difficult pathology of the wrist, with particular emphasis on management based on staging.

Asif M. Ilyas, MD
Hand and Upper Extremity Surgery
Rothman Institute
Thomas Jefferson University
925 Chestnut Street
Philadelphia, PA 19107, USA

E-mail address:
asif.ilyas@rothmaninstitute.com

orthopedic.theclinics.com

The Management of Type II Superior Labral Anterior to Posterior Injuries

Frank McCormick, MD[a],[*], Sanjeev Bhatia, MD[b],
Peter Chalmers, MD[b], Anil Gupta, MD, MBA[b],
Nikhil Verma, MD[b], Anthony A. Romeo, MD[b]

KEYWORDS

- Superior labrum anterior to posterior tears • Biceps tenodesis • Arthroscopic repair
- Type II SLAP tear

KEY POINTS

- Superior labral anterior to posterior (SLAP) repair failure is unclear and likely multifactorial.
- Current evidence offers no consensus on the dynamic muscular role of the long head of the biceps tendon in the glenohumeral joint.
- SLAP repairs result in slightly higher outcomes but at an increased complication rate and rehabilitation.
- Arthroscopic SLAP repairs remain the gold standard; however, clinicians are cautious in older patients and overhead athletes.
- The authors recommend tenodesis in the revision setting.

INTRODUCTION

Superior labral anterior to posterior (SLAP) tears were first recognized by Andrews and colleagues[1] nearly 30 years ago in throwing athletes.[2] Snyder and colleagues[3] later classified these injuries into 4 basic subtypes.

Type I lesions are characterized by fraying at the inner margin of the labrum, which can be

Funding Sources: The authors did not receive any outside funding or grants in support of their research for or preparation of this work. Neither they nor a member of their immediate families received payments or other benefits or a commitment or agreement to provide such benefits from a commercial entity.
Conflicts of Interest: Not related to this work, Dr A.A. Romeo has a financial relationship with the following entities: speakers bureau member for Arthrex Inc. and DJO Surgical; consultant for Arthrex Inc.; receives grant/research support from DJO Surgical, Ossur, and Smith & Nephew plc; and receives royalties from Arthrex Inc. Not related to this work, Dr N. Verma has a financial relationship with the following entities: board member of Smith & Nephew plc, Shoulder Advisory Board, and Vindico Medical Education; consultant for Smith & Nephew plc; receives grant/research support from Arthroscopy Association of North America and Major League Baseball; receives royalties from Smith & Nephew plc; has stock/stock options at Omeros Corporation; and receives fellowship and research support from Arthrex Inc., Smith & Nephew plc, Ossur, and ConMed Linvatec. Drs F. McCormick, S. Bhatia, P. Chalmers, and A. Gupta, their immediate families, and any research foundation with which they are affiliated, did not receive any financial payments or other benefits from any commercial entity related to the subject of this article.
The enclosed work has been read and approved by all authors. No information in this article has been published elsewhere as part of other work. Each author believes that the article represents honest work.
[a] Midwest Orthopaedics at Rush, Rush University Medical Center, 1611 West Harrison Street, Suite 300, Chicago, IL 60612, USA; [b] Division of Sports Medicine, Department of Orthopedic Surgery, Rush University Medical Center, Rush Medical College of Rush University, 1611 West Harrison Street, Suite 300, Chicago, IL 60612, USA
* Corresponding author.
E-mail address: drfrankmccormick@yahoo.com

Orthop Clin N Am 45 (2014) 121–128
http://dx.doi.org/10.1016/j.ocl.2013.08.008
0030-5898/14/$ – see front matter © 2014 Elsevier Inc. All rights reserved.

considered a normal part of the aging process.[2] Type II lesions are the most common variant, consisting of a separation of the biceps and labrum from the superior glenoid, erythema at the SLAP anchor insertion, and a minimum of 5 mm of excursion (**Fig. 1**).[3] A sulcus of 1 to 2 mm is considered normal.[4] Intraoperatively placing the arm in abduction and external rotation and arthroscopically observing the peel-back phenomenon can confirm the diagnosis.[5] Type II SLAP lesions have also been further subclassified into anterior, posterior, and combined, wherein the direction of tear propagation progresses to concomitant directional microinstability and partial-thickness rotator cuff tears (ie, posterior extension predicted posterior microinstability and posterior partial rotator cuff tears).[6] Type III lesions are characterized by an intact biceps complex junction at the superior glenoid but with a bucket-handle–type tear within the superior labral complex. A type IV tear is a type III tear with a concomitant separation of the superolabral junction with the glenoid, thus, also meeting the diagnosis of a type II lesion.

Maffet and colleagues[7] expanded the original classification to include type V through VII lesions. Type V lesions are SLAP lesions in continuity with anteroinferior Bankart-type labral lesions and type VI lesions involve biceps tendon separation with an unstable flap of the labrum. In type VII lesions, the superior-labrum biceps tendon separation extends below the middle glenohumeral ligament.

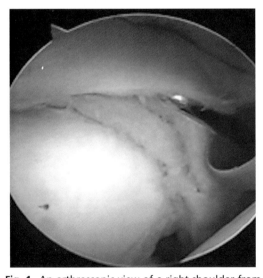

Fig. 1. An arthroscopic view of a right shoulder from the posterior portal in the beach chair position shows a type II superior labral tear with complete separation of the biceps labral junction from the glenoid. An intraoperative peel-back sign with the arm in 90° of abduction with external rotation was confirmatory.

SLAP tears have been further characterized into 10 subtypes based on concurrent instability and posterior extension.[8]

The optimal management of patients with suspected SLAP tears remains controversial. At a minimum, patients should undergo 3 months of conservative management before surgical options are explored. Conservative treatment begins with rest, activity modification, and oral anti-inflammatory prescriptions. A formal physical therapy protocol should be instituted to address any scapular dyskinesis and rotator cuff imbalance with open and closed chain exercises. Stretching of the posterior capsule via the sleeper stretch may also be effective. If these initial measures are successful, the authors advance therapy to include core and trunk strengthening, followed by a formal throwing protocol.

The incidence of surgically treated SLAP tears has risen dramatically over the past decade.[9,10] Arthroscopic repair of type II SLAP tears that have failed to respond to conservative treatment is currently the standard of care. Numerous prospective trials have shown good to excellent surgical outcomes at 2-year follow-up (**Table 1**).[11–13] Furthermore, a recent meta-analysis of outcomes after arthroscopic surgical repair of type II SLAP lesions showed that 83% of patients had good-to-excellent satisfaction scores and 73% of athletes returned to their preinjury level of play.

Despite the overall good to excellent outcomes and high patient satisfaction, challenges remain in the care of these lesions in overhead athletes, older patients, and patients who develop postoperative stiffness. Functional results of overhead athletes are inferior to those of the general population; on average, one-third of overhead athletes are unable to return to their previous level of function after SLAP repair.[14] Postoperative stiffness is the most common complication. Most patients require 6 months to regain full range of motion. In addition, up to one-fifth of patients lack full range of motion 5 years postoperatively. For instance, in a large prospective series involving military patients, mean forward flexion and external rotation were significantly reduced at final follow-up.[11] Older patients also tend to have significantly worse functional results.[11,15,16]

Biceps tenodesis has been proposed as a surgical alternative, particularly in older patients and overhead athletes.[16] Biceps tenodesis has a low complication rate, a high rate of postoperative patient satisfaction, and excellent functional outcomes. This article discusses the role of biceps tenodesis in the management of SLAP tears.

Table 1
A comparison of prospective studies of arthroscopic type II SLAP repairs with a minimum 2-year follow-up reported in the literature

Study	Enrollment	ASES Mean[a]	Standard Deviation	Mean Follow-up
Provencher et al,[11] 2013	179	88.2	5.3	40.4
Denard et al,[15] 2012	55	86.2	NR	77.0
Brockmeier et al,[12] 2009	47	97.0	10.8	32.4
Friel et al,[13] 2010	48	83.3	NR	40.8
Silberberg et al,[53] 2011	32	93.9	13.0	37.0

Abbreviation: NR, not reported.
[a] The average ASES score of 361 patients undergoing repair is 88.8.

CAUSES OF FAILURE OF SLAP REPAIR

Surgical repair of type II SLAP lesions involves arthroscopic fixations of the labrum and biceps insertion to the superior glenoid.[17,18] A variety of techniques have been devised for this anatomic repair, including suture anchor and bioabsorbable tack fixation. Irrespective of techniques, common causes of failure are recognized (**Fig. 2**). Postoperative stiffness can be caused by intraoperative technical errors. Inadvertent restriction of physiologic biceps excursion from overtensioning the repair or from nonanatomic biceps anchor reduction can contribute to this. Overhead athletes are particularly prone to this complication. Sutures placed anterior to the biceps into the rotator interval tissue can lead to overtensioning of the anterior capsule, superior glenohumeral ligament, and even middle glenohumeral ligament, which can result in loss of external rotation (**Fig. 3**).

Intraoperative complications can include suture anchor pullout, suture granuloma formation, suture pullout, synovitis, glenoid osteochondrolysis from prominent hardware, suprascapular nerve injury from medial anchor placement, and a delaminated long head of the biceps.[16,19–25]

SLAP repair failure may also be related to failure of the labrum to heal to the superior glenoid. The anterior-superior labrum and glenoid are devoid of vascular supply, particularly near the attachment of the biceps root, which may limit healing potential.[26] This healing interface is subject to shear forces, friction, traction, and pressure during physiologic shoulder range of motion, propagating tendon degeneration, and pain.[19,27] Rotator cuff

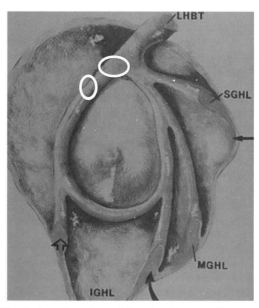

Fig. 3. A en face view of the glenoid shows the proximity of the superior glenohumeral and middle glenohumeral ligaments to the biceps-labral complex. A SLAP repair has the potential to tighten these ligaments, leading to postoperative stiffness. The authors prefer to place the anchors primarily posterior to the biceps (*right circle*), and may add another anchor if the tear propagates posteriorly (*left circle*).

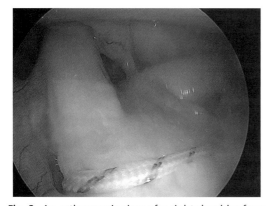

Fig. 2. An arthroscopic view of a right shoulder from the posterior portal in the lateral position shows a failed type II superior labral tear. Loose sutures and anterior rotator interval synovitis are common findings, with the clear cause of failure often unknown. A subpectoral biceps tenodesis was performed.

dysfunction with associated proximal migration of the humeral head may amplify these stresses. As shown by Refior and Sowa,[27] these stresses on the tendon are most notably present when cuff dysfunction (eg, tendonitis, partial- or full-thickness tears) is concomitant. In addition, patients may experience persistent pain despite healing because the proximal, intra-articular portion of the long head of the biceps tendon (LHBT) contains sensory and sympathetic fibers that may be involved in the pathogenesis of shoulder pain.[28]

THE BIOMECHANICAL AND CLINICAL FUNCTION OF THE BICEPS

LHBT has a unique anatomic course, traveling through the intertubercular groove before making a 30° turn to become intra-articular and attach at the supraglenoid tubercle and superior labrum. The biceps primarily functions as an elbow flexor and forearm supinator. The function of the LHBT within the glenohumeral joint is largely unknown, and understanding of this function is crucial for determining the proper treatment for abnormalities of the biceps anchor, intra-articular biceps, biceps pulley, and intertubercular biceps. Some argue that the tendon does not play a role in glenohumeral stability, humeral migration, or glenohumeral function. If this is true, then tenodesis could be appropriate in the treatment of SLAP tears in nearly all settings. Strongly supporting this argument is the almost complete lack of glenohumeral instability, proximal humeral migration, or functional deficit in patient's status after tenodesis.[29,30]

The LHBT may play a role as a secondary glenohumeral stabilizer. Cadaveric resection of the LHBT increases anterior and inferior humeral translation in adduction[31–34] and increases strain within the inferior glenohumeral ligament.[35] Conversely, axial traction placed on the LHBT decreases glenohumeral laxity.[36] Electromyographic function within the LHBT is increased in patients with rotator cuff tears.[37]

However, equally convincing evidence suggests that the LHBT may play no role as a secondary glenohumeral stabilizer. Cadaveric studies in which the SLAP tears were created without violation of the superior or middle glenohumeral ligaments show no change in glenohumeral laxity.[38,39] In addition, patients with anterior instability with activities of daily living have decreased LHBT electromyographic function, suggested reflex latency, and a role as a glenohumeral destabilizer.[40] These electromyographic findings have been replicated in pitchers with instability.[41,42] In summary, the current evidence offers no consensus on the role of the LHBT as a secondary glenohumeral stabilizer.

The LHBT may also play a role as a humeral head depressor. Cadaveric evidence suggests that resection of the LHBT causes proximal humeral migration.[43] Fluoroscopically, proximal humeral migration has been observed in patients with SLAP tears.[44] However, clinically, no proximal humeral migration has been observed after tenodesis.[16,29,30] The current evidence thus offers no consensus on the role of the LHBT as a humeral depressor.

The LHBT may play a dynamic muscular role in glenohumeral function. Clinically, continued electromyographic function within the LHBT has been demonstrated with elbow and forearm immobilization.[45] However, other authors have shown conflicting findings using a similar experimental model examining LHBT electromyographic function during elbow and forearm immobilization.[46] A study examining patterns of electromyographic activity in the rotator cuff, deltoid, biceps, and adductors showed desynchronization of the biceps from the remainder of these muscles, suggesting that the biceps does not play a role in coordinated glenohumeral function.[47] The current evidence thus offers no consensus on the dynamic muscular role of the LHBT in the glenohumeral joint. In unpublished work in a cadaveric model, the authors were unable to show any effect of SLAP tears or biceps tenodesis on glenohumeral stability.

CLINICAL COMPARISON OF BICEPS TENODESIS AND SLAP REPAIR

Given the lack of a clear biomechanical or clinical need for the long head of the biceps insertion into the glenohumeral joint, the authors compared clinical outcomes and complications of SLAP repair and biceps tenodesis. The prospective trials have a total of 361 patients. All studies presented the American Shoulder and Elbow Surgeons (ASES) patient-reported outcome score, which has been shown to be reliable, responsive, and valid, with a minimal clinically important difference (MCID) of 6.4.[48,49] Mean ASES score after SLAP repair was 88.8. These outcomes parallel results of a recent meta-analysis, which showed 83% good-to-excellent patient satisfaction.[14]

In comparison, fewer published series have examined clinical outcomes of biceps tenodesis. A recent systematic review of biceps tenotomy and tenodesis[50] concluded a 74% good to excellent outcome; an 8% cosmetic deformity rate with tenodesis versus a tenotomy's 79% good to excellent outcome; and a 38% cosmetic deformity rate. **Table 2** lists the mean ASES scores for surgeries in which the LHBT was removed from its

Table 2
Comparison of identified studies that surgically removed the long head of the biceps from the superior labrum and reported ASES outcome score

Study	Enrollment	ASES Mean[a]	Standard Deviation	Mean Follow-up[b]
Mazzocca et al,[54] 2008	50	81.0	NR	29
Gill et al,[52] 2001	30	81.8	NR	19
Drakos et al,[55] 2008	40	84.8	NR	28
Millett et al,[38] 2008	88	76.0	NR	13

Abbreviation: NR, not reported.
[a] Summing the biceps tenodesis, tenotomy, or transfer scores, the mean ASES score is 79.7 in 208 patients.
[b] Most patients did not meet 24 months' follow-up.

insertion (tenotomy/tenodesis/transfer). The mean ASES score is 79.7, which is a clinically and statistically significant difference compared with the SLAP repair outcomes (P<.0001), conceding a heterogeneous patient population. This finding indicates an outcome advantage for SLAP repairs over biceps tenotomy/tenodesis/transfers, because it represents an ASES difference greater than the MCID of 6.4. However, with the known risk factors of advanced age and workers' compensation status, the comparative advantage diminishes below the expected clinical difference, yet imparts a longer recovery with greater risk of complications. Compared with the aforementioned SLAP repair complication rate, biceps tenodesis presents limited surgical morbidity. Over a 3-year period at the authors' institution, 373 biceps tenodeses were performed, with only 8 complications: 2 patients (0.18%) with persistent bicipital pain; 2 patients (0.18%) with failure of fixation Popeye

deformity; 1 patient (0.09%) with deep wound infection; 1 patient (0.09%) with temporary neuropathy; 1 patient (0.09%) with reflex sympathetic dystrophy; and 1 patient (0.09%) with proximal humerus fracture.[51] Moreover, a biceps tenodesis requires a less formal rehabilitation, often with a return to work at 6 to 8 weeks. Gill and colleagues[52] report a 97% rate of return to work at 2 weeks with a simple tenotomy. To many patients, the possible marginal clinical benefit of a SLAP repair may not be worth the protracted rehabilitation and increased risk for complications. A full discussion with patients regarding the advantages and disadvantages of both procedures can be helpful in surgical decision making (**Fig. 4**).

CURRENT TREATMENT RECOMMENDATIONS

The current standard of care for a type II SLAP lesion that has failed conservative management

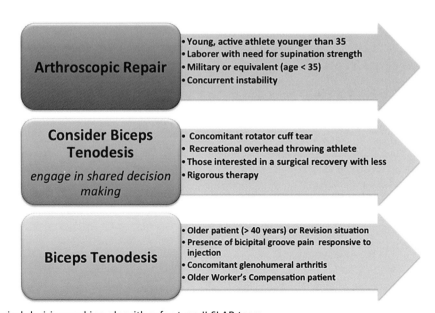

Arthroscopic Repair
- Young, active athlete younger than 35
- Laborer with need for supination strength
- Military or equivalent (age < 35)
- Concurrent instability

Consider Biceps Tenodesis
engage in shared decision making
- Concomitant rotator cuff tear
- Recreational overhead throwing athlete
- Those interested in a surgical recovery with less
- Rigorous therapy

Biceps Tenodesis
- Older patient (> 40 years) or Revision situation
- Presence of bicipital groove pain responsive to injection
- Concomitant glenohumeral arthritis
- Older Worker's Compensation patient

Fig. 4. Surgical decision-making algorithm for type II SLAP tears.

is an arthroscopic repair using bioabsorbable anchors with nonabsorbable sutures. With this approach, most patients can expect good to excellent results. However, biceps tenodesis may offer superior outcomes in a select group of patients, namely older patients, workers' compensation patients, and those wishing to avoid increased surgical risk with a protracted rehabilitation course at the expense of optimal function.

Surgical treatment of the overhead athlete is less clear. After SLAP repair, these athletes have a 65% rate of return to their previous level of play. Poor return to play may be more a function of throwing mechanics than surgical repair. In the young throwing athlete, the authors recommend arthroscopic repair with anchors. However, patient expectations must be appropriately managed with a full preoperative discussion regarding return to play rates. In particular, one series involving older overhead athletes showed superior return-to-play rates after biceps tenodesis compared with SLAP repair.[16] Whether these results can be extrapolated to younger athletes remains unclear. If additional biomechanical data confirm the lack of a glenohumeral function for the long head of the biceps, surgeons may feel more inclined to remove the tendon from the potentially pain-generating bicipital groove. However, given the potential role of the LHBT as a secondary glenohumeral stabilizer, tenodesis should be considered with caution as the primary treatment for type II SLAP lesions in overhead throwing athletes. The authors recommend a biceps tenodesis in the setting of SLAP tear revision surgery.

REFERENCES

1. Andrews JR, Carson WG Jr, McLeod WD. Glenoid labrum tears related to the long head of the biceps. Am J Sports Med 1985;13(5):337–41.
2. Pfahler M, Haraida S, Schulz C, et al. Age-related changes of the glenoid labrum in normal shoulders. J Shoulder Elbow Surg 2003;12(1):40–52.
3. Snyder SJ, Karzel RP, Del Pizzo W, et al. SLAP lesions of the shoulder. Arthroscopy 1990;6(4):274–9.
4. Rao AG, Kim TK, Chronopoulos E, et al. Anatomical variants in the anterosuperior aspect of the glenoid labrum: a statistical analysis of seventy-three cases. J Bone Joint Surg Am 2003;85(4):653–9.
5. Burkhart SS, Morgan CD. The peel-back mechanism: its role in producing and extending posterior type II SLAP lesions and its effect on SLAP repair rehabilitation. Arthroscopy 1998;14(6):637–40.
6. Morgan CD, Burkhart SS, Palmeri M, et al. Type II SLAP lesions: three subtypes and their relationships to superior instability and rotator cuff tears. Arthroscopy 1998;14(6):553–65.
7. Maffet MW, Gartsman GM, Moseley B. Superior labrum-biceps tendon complex lesions of the shoulder. Am J Sports Med 1995;23(1):93–8.
8. Powell S, Nord KD, Ryu RK. The diagnosis, classification, and treatment of SLAP Lesions. Oper Tech Sports Med 2004;12(2):99–110.
9. Weber SC, Martin DF, Seiler JG 3rd, et al. Superior labrum anterior and posterior lesions of the shoulder: incidence rates, complications, and outcomes as reported by American Board of Orthopedic Surgery part II candidates. Am J Sports Med 2012; 40(7):1538–43.
10. Zhang AL, Kreulen C, Ngo SS, et al. Demographic trends in arthroscopic SLAP repair in the United States. Am J Sports Med 2012;40(5):1144–7.
11. Provencher MT, McCormick F, Dewing CB, et al. A prospective analysis of 179 type 2 superior labrum anterior and posterior repairs: outcomes and factors associated with success and failure. Am J Sports Med 2013;41(4):880–6.
12. Brockmeier SF, Voos JE, Williams RJ 3rd, et al. Outcomes after arthroscopic repair of type-II SLAP lesions. J Bone Joint Surg Am 2009;91(7): 1595–603.
13. Friel NA, Karas V, Slabaugh MA, et al. Outcomes of type II superior labrum, anterior to posterior (SLAP) repair: prospective evaluation at a minimum two-year follow-up. J Shoulder Elbow Surg 2010; 19(6):859–67.
14. Sayde WM, Cohen SB, Ciccotti MG, et al. Return to play after type II superior labral anterior-posterior lesion repairs in athletes: a systematic review. Clin Orthop Relat Res 2012;470(6):1595–600.
15. Denard PJ, Ladermann A, Burkhart SS. Long-term outcome after arthroscopic repair of type II SLAP lesions: results according to age and workers' compensation status. Arthroscopy 2012;28(4): 451–7.
16. Boileau P, Parratte S, Chuinard C, et al. Arthroscopic treatment of isolated type II SLAP lesions: biceps tenodesis as an alternative to reinsertion. Am J Sports Med 2009;37(5):929–36.
17. Neuman BJ, Boisvert CB, Reiter B, et al. Results of arthroscopic repair of type II superior labral anterior posterior lesions in overhead athletes: assessment of return to preinjury playing level and satisfaction. Am J Sports Med 2011;39(9):1883–8.
18. Uggen C, Wei A, Glousman RE, et al. Biomechanical comparison of knotless anchor repair versus simple suture repair for type II SLAP lesions. Arthroscopy 2009;25(10):1085–92.
19. Byram IR, Dunn WR, Kuhn JE. Humeral head abrasion: an association with failed superior labrum anterior posterior repairs. J Shoulder Elbow Surg 2011;20(1):92–7.
20. Cohen DB, Coleman S, Drakos MC, et al. Outcomes of isolated type II SLAP lesions treated

20. with arthroscopic fixation using a bioabsorbable tack. Arthroscopy 2006;22(2):136–42.

21. Ifesanya A, Scheibel M. Posterosuperior suture granuloma impingement after arthroscopic SLAP repair using suture anchors: a case report. Knee Surg Sports Traumatol Arthrosc 2008;16(7):703–6.

22. Park S, Glousman RE. Outcomes of revision arthroscopic type II superior labral anterior posterior repairs. Am J Sports Med 2011;39(6):1290–4.

23. Sassmannshausen G, Sukay M, Mair SD. Broken or dislodged poly-L-lactic acid bioabsorbable tacks in patients after SLAP lesion surgery. Arthroscopy 2006;22(6):615–9.

24. Kim SH, Koh YG, Sung CH, et al. Iatrogenic suprascapular nerve injury after repair of type II SLAP lesion. Arthroscopy 2010;26(7):1005–8.

25. Saltzman M, Mercer D, Bertelsen A, et al. Postsurgical chondrolysis of the shoulder. Orthopedics 2009;32(3):215.

26. Abrassart S, Stern R, Hoffmeyer P. Arterial supply of the glenoid: an anatomic study. J Shoulder Elbow Surg 2006;15(2):232–8.

27. Refior HJ, Sowa D. Long tendon of the biceps brachii: sites of predilection for degenerative lesions. J Shoulder Elbow Surg 1995;4(6):436–40.

28. Alpantaki K, McLaughlin D, Karagogeos D, et al. Sympathetic and sensory neural elements in the tendon of the long head of the biceps. J Bone Joint Surg Am 2005;87(7):1580–3.

29. Boileau P, Baque F, Valerio L, et al. Isolated arthroscopic biceps tenotomy or tenodesis improves symptoms in patients with massive irreparable rotator cuff tears. J Bone Joint Surg Am 2007;89(4):747–57.

30. Boileau P, Krishnan SG, Coste JS, et al. Arthroscopic biceps tenodesis: a new technique using bioabsorbable interference screw fixation. Arthroscopy 2002;18(9):1002–12.

31. McMahon PJ, Burkart A, Musahl V, et al. Glenohumeral translations are increased after a type II superior labrum anterior-posterior lesion: a cadaveric study of severity of passive stabilizer injury. J Shoulder Elbow Surg 2004;13(1):39–44.

32. Mihata T, McGarry MH, Tibone JE, et al. Biomechanical assessment of Type II superior labral anterior-posterior (SLAP) lesions associated with anterior shoulder capsular laxity as seen in throwers: a cadaveric study. Am J Sports Med 2008;36(8):1604–10.

33. Panossian VR, Mihata T, Tibone JE, et al. Biomechanical analysis of isolated type II SLAP lesions and repair. J Shoulder Elbow Surg 2005;14(5):529–34.

34. Burkart A, Debski RE, Musahl V, et al. Glenohumeral translations are only partially restored after repair of a simulated type II superior labral lesion. Am J Sports Med 2003;31(1):56–63.

35. Rodosky MW, Harner CD, Fu FH. The role of the long head of the biceps muscle and superior glenoid labrum in anterior stability of the shoulder. Am J Sports Med 1994;22(1):121–30.

36. Pagnani MJ, Deng XH, Warren RF, et al. Role of the long head of the biceps brachii in glenohumeral stability: a biomechanical study in cadavera. J Shoulder Elbow Surg 1996;5(4):255–62.

37. Kido T, Itoi E, Konno N, et al. Electromyographic activities of the biceps during arm elevation in shoulders with rotator cuff tears. Acta Orthop Scand 1998;69(6):575–9.

38. Millett PJ, Sanders B, Gobezie R, et al. Interference screw vs. suture anchor fixation for open subpectoral biceps tenodesis: does it matter? BMC Musculoskelet Disord 2008;9:121.

39. Youm T, Tibone JE, ElAttrache NS, et al. Simulated type II superior labral anterior posterior lesions do not alter the path of glenohumeral articulation: a cadaveric biomechanical study. Am J Sports Med 2008;36(4):767–74.

40. Myers JB, Ju YY, Hwang JH, et al. Reflexive muscle activation alterations in shoulders with anterior glenohumeral instability. Am J Sports Med 2004;32(4):1013–21.

41. Glousman R, Jobe F, Tibone J, et al. Dynamic electromyographic analysis of the throwing shoulder with glenohumeral instability. J Bone Joint Surg Am 1988;70(2):220–6.

42. Illyes A, Kiss RM. Electromyographic analysis in patients with multidirectional shoulder instability during pull, forward punch, elevation and overhead throw. Knee Surg Sports Traumatol Arthrosc 2007;15(5):624–31.

43. Kumar VP, Satku K, Balasubramaniam P. The role of the long head of biceps brachii in the stabilization of the head of the humerus. Clin Orthop Relat Res 1989;(244):172–5.

44. Warner JJ, McMahon PJ. The role of the long head of the biceps brachii in superior stability of the glenohumeral joint. J Bone Joint Surg Am 1995;77(3):366–72.

45. Sakurai G, Ozaki J, Tomita Y, et al. Electromyographic analysis of shoulder joint function of the biceps brachii muscle during isometric contraction. Clin Orthop Relat Res 1998;(354):123–31.

46. Yamaguchi K, Riew KD, Galatz LM, et al. Biceps activity during shoulder motion: an electromyographic analysis. Clin Orthop Relat Res 1997;(336):122–9.

47. Hawkes DH, Alizadehkhaiyat O, Fisher AC, et al. Normal shoulder muscular activation and coordination during a shoulder elevation task based on activities of daily living: an electromyographic study. J Orthop Res 2012;30(1):53–60.

48. Michener LA, McClure PW, Sennett BJ. American Shoulder and Elbow Surgeons Standardized

Shoulder Assessment Form, patient self-report section: reliability, validity, and responsiveness. J Shoulder Elbow Surg 2002;11(6):587–94.

49. Roy JS, MacDermid JC, Woodhouse LJ. Measuring shoulder function: a systematic review of four questionnaires. Arthritis Rheum 2009;61(5):623–32.

50. Slenker NR, Lawson K, Ciccotti MG, et al. Biceps tenotomy versus tenodesis: clinical outcomes. Arthroscopy 2012;28(4):576–82.

51. Nho SJ, Reiff SN, Verma NN, et al. Complications associated with subpectoral biceps tenodesis: low rates of incidence following surgery. J Shoulder Elbow Surg 2010;19(5):764–8.

52. Gill TJ, McIrvin E, Mair SD, et al. Results of biceps tenotomy for treatment of pathology of the long head of the biceps brachii. J Shoulder Elbow Surg 2001;10(3):247–9.

53. Silberberg JM, Moya-Angeler J, Martin E, et al. Vertical versus horizontal suture configuration for the repair of isolated type II SLAP lesion through a single anterior portal: a randomized controlled trial. Arthroscopy 2011;27(12):1605–13.

54. Mazzocca AD, Cote MP, Arciero CL, et al. Clinical outcomes after subpectoral biceps tenodesis with an interference screw. Am J Sports Med 2008; 36(10):1922–9.

55. Drakos MC, Verma NN, Gulotta LV, et al. Arthroscopic transfer of the long head of the biceps tendon: functional outcome and clinical results. Arthroscopy 2008;24(2):217–23.

Carpal Instability of the Wrist

Nicholas Caggiano, MD[a], Kristofer S. Matullo, MD[b,c],*

KEYWORDS

- Carpal tunnel • Wrist • Instability • Ligaments

KEY POINTS

- The dorsal aspect of the scapholunate ligament is the strongest of its 3 subregions.
- The common mechanism of injury to the scapholunate and lunotriquetral ligaments is extension, ulnar deviation, and intercarpal supination.
- Although scapholunate widening on a posteroanterior view of the wrist indicates scapholunate ligament injury, this is not a sensitive finding, and continued complaints of pain and/or instability should warrant further work-up.
- Arthroscopic debridement is an appropriate treatment of partial tears.
- Repair should be attempted for acute tears.
- Reconstruction can be attempted for chronic tears that remain reducible.
- Salvage options can be offered for irreducible injuries or in cases with degenerative changes.

INTRODUCTION

Injuries to the scapholunate and lunotriquetral ligaments can have severe deleterious effects. The scaphoid acts as a connecting rod between the proximal and distal rows.[1] The scaphoid is tethered directly by the scapholunate ligament and indirectly by the lunotriquetral ligament. Disruption of these stabilizing ligaments leads to abnormal mechanics of the carpal joints. Both the quality of reduction and the timing of definitive management affect outcomes following dissociative carpal instability. This article explains the anatomy, biomechanics, mechanism of injury, studies, and treatment algorithms involved in caring for patients with dissociative carpal instability.

ANATOMY

The carpal bones are divided into 2 U-shaped rows: the proximal row containing the scaphoid, lunate, triquetrum, and pisiform; and the distal row, which is composed of the trapezium, trapezoid, capitate, and hamate. Both intrinsic and extrinsic ligaments connect the two rows. These ligaments are generally characterized as either palmar or dorsal and are often described as thickenings of the joint capsule.

Of the intrinsic ligaments of the wrist, the most important for stability are the scapholunate and lunotriquetral interosseous ligaments. The scapholunate ligament is a C-shaped ligament composed of dorsal, central, and palmar subregions. These three subregions attach at their respective articular margins of the scaphoid and lunate.

The dorsal subregion of the scapholunate ligament consists of transversely oriented collagen fibers. This dorsal aspect is the strongest and thickest of the three subregions and provides the greatest contribution to the stability of the scapholunate articulation.[2] The central subregion is thinner than the dorsal component and is obliquely oriented, in contrast with the transverse fibers of the dorsal component. The central subregion is not considered a true ligament but more a fibrocartilaginous structure. It merges with the dorsal aspect of the scapholunate ligament, but is separated from the volar subregion by the volar radioscapholunate ligament

[a] Department of Orthopaedic Surgery, St. Luke's University Hospital, 801 Ostrum Street, PPH-2, Bethlehem, PA 18015, USA; [b] Division of Hand Surgery, St. Luke's University Hospital and Health Network, 801 Ostrum Street, PPH-2, Bethlehem, PA 18015, USA; [c] Department of Orthopaedic Surgery, Temple University Hospital, 3401 Broad Street, Philadelphia, PA 19140, USA

* Corresponding author. Department of Orthopaedic Surgery, PPH2, 801 Ostrum Street, Bethlehem, PA 18015.
E-mail address: kristofer.matullo@sluhn.org

Orthop Clin N Am 45 (2014) 129–140
http://dx.doi.org/10.1016/j.ocl.2013.08.009
0030-5898/14/$ – see front matter © 2014 Elsevier Inc. All rights reserved.

(ligament of Testut).[2] The volar region of the scapholunate ligament is a thin (often less than 1 mm thick)[2] layer composed of obliquely oriented fibers. These fibers are confluent with the radioscapholunate ligament proximally and are sometimes seen to be interconnected with the radioscaphocapitate ligament distally. A sharp division exists palmarly between the volar region and the long radiolunate ligament. The volar region is thought to function as a ligament, but does not confer as much stability to the scapholunate ligament as does the dorsal region.

Additional stabilizers to the scapholunate joint exist on the palmar and dorsal sides of the wrist. The scaphotrapeziotrapezoid and scaphocapitate ligaments lie on the dorsal aspect and provide resistance against the tendency of the scaphoid to palmar flex. The radioscaphocapitate and short and long radiolunate ligaments lend stability on the palmar side of the wrist.[3]

The lunotriquetral ligament is also composed of 3 subregions, 2 true ligaments on the dorsal and palmar aspects and a fibrocartilaginous central segment, similar to the scapholunate ligament. The relative strengths of the three subregions are opposite to those of the scapholunate ligament, with the volar aspect being the thickest and the greatest contributor to lunotriquetral stability.

The proximal carpal row has no tendinous insertion, and is thus often termed the intercalated segment. Three sets of tendons cross the proximal row: the extrinsic flexors and extensors of the fingers; the flexors and extensors of the wrist; and the abductor pollicis longus and the extensor pollicis brevis, which course around the radial styloid. Movement between the carpal bones is negligible. Because there are no muscular attachments onto the proximal carpal row, the movement of the proximal row carpal bones is determined by their ligamentous attachments and the mechanical forces of the tendons that cross the wrist.[4]

BIOMECHANICS

Because the proximal carpal row has no tendinous insertion, the forces that act on its proximal and distal articular surfaces dictate the forces that act on the intercalated segment. The tendons that cross the proximal row exert a compressive force that is resisted by the connecting-rod action of the scaphoid. Instability of the scaphoid leads to an alteration of the articulation between the proximal and distal rows.

During radial deviation of the normal wrist, the trapezoid and trapezium exert a volarly directed force on the distal pole of the scaphoid. This force causes the scaphoid to flex about its waist; this flexion force is then transmitted to the lunate via

the scapholunate ligament and to the trapezium via the lunotriquetral ligament. The proximal row radially deviates as 1 unit.[5]

Ulnar deviation of the normal wrist causes the hamate to project a dorsally directed force on the triquetrum. As the triquetrum is rotated dorsally by the hamate, a competent lunotriquetral ligament imparts an extension moment on the lunate, and indirectly on the scaphoid via the scapholunate ligament. It is through this mechanism that ulnar deviation causes extension of the wrist.[5]

The lunate can be thought of as existing in a balanced suspension between the scaphoid and the triquetrum. The scaphoid has a flexion bias, and through the scapholunate ligament exerts a flexion moment on the lunate. However, the triquetrum has an extension bias, and exerts an extension moment on the lunate through the lunotriquetral ligament. In a balanced proximal carpal row, the lunate remains centered on the distal radius without tilting into flexion or extension. The tendons that cross the wrist exert a compressive force across the carpus through the centrally located capitate at the capitolunate articulation.

In the uninjured wrist, the lunate is held in a tightly coupled balance between the scaphoid and the triquetrum. However, injury to either the scapholunate ligament or the lunotriquetral ligament causes respective extension or flexion of the lunate. With disruption of the scapholunate ligament, a gap opens between the scaphoid and the lunate, into which the capitate eventually collapses. The scaphoid, now free of its tether to the lunate, assumes a position of flexion as the capitate comes to occupy the distal space between the lunate and the scaphoid. The lunate, no longer balanced by the flexion moment from the scaphoid, is rotated into extension by the triquetrum. The lunate angles dorsally, producing the pattern known as dorsal intercalated segment instability (DISI).

Unlike injury to the scapholunate ligament, isolated injury of the lunotriquetral ligament is rarely sufficient to allow the flexion moment of the scaphoid to palmar flex the lunate.[6] However, if the dorsal radiocarpal ligament is also injured, the tethering effect on the dorsum of the lunate is lost and the scaphoid and lunate angle into flexion while the capitate begins to migrate between the lunate and the triquetrum.[1] Thus, injury to both the lunotriquetral and dorsal radiocarpal ligaments leads to volar intercalated segment instability (VISI).

MECHANISM OF INJURY AND CLASSIFICATION

Injury to the scapholunate or lunotriquetral ligaments is most commonly caused by a fall on an outstretched hand. Other common causes include sports injuries and high-energy trauma such as motor vehicle collisions. Mayfield and colleagues[7] were able to reproduce scapholunate injuries via direct impact to the hypothenar region with the wrist in extension, ulnar deviation, and intercarpal supination. These types of trauma can lead to a spectrum of injuries, including injury to the ligaments of the wrist, fracture of the distal radius, and even fracture of one or more carpal bones depending on the angle of the carpus when the impact occurs.[8,9]

Dissociative carpal instability is often directly caused by hyperextension of the wrist. Mayfield and colleagues[7] proposed that a continuum of injuries occur about the wrist with extension, ulnar deviation, and carpal supination. They described a 4-part circular progression of injury, which they termed progressive perilunar instability (PLI) as follows (**Fig. 1**):

- Stage I: dorsal migration of the proximal pole of the scaphoid with resulting injury to the scapholunate ligament.
- Stage II: further extension, ulnar deviation, and supination of the carpus leads to progression of the force through the space of Poirier.
- Stage III: progression of these forces causes the triquetrum to translate away from the lunate with resultant injury to the lunotriquetral ligament.
- Stage IV: disruption of the dorsal radiocarpal ligament allows the lunate to rotate on its

palmar ligamentous hinge and dislocate with resultant articulation of the capitate into the lunate facet of the distal radius.

Mayfield and colleagues'[7] model has often been cited in the literature as an explanation of the progression of scapholunate injury through perilunate dislocation, lunotriquetral disruption, and eventually to lunate dislocation. However, this model does not explain an isolated lunotriquetral ligament injury without concomitant scapholunate injury.

A mechanism opposite to that of Mayfield and colleagues[7] was recently proposed to explain ulnar-sided injuries of the wrist. Shin and colleagues[6] investigated isolated lunotriquetral injuries to the ulnar side of the wrist caused by fall, twisting, or sports. Subsequent cadaveric testing led to a description of a 3-stage mechanism for ulnar-sided injury to the wrist leading to dorsal perilunate dislocation. The model is as follows:

- Stage I: disruption of the lunotriquetral ligament
- Stage II: stage I plus disruption of the ulnolunate, ulnotriquetral, ulnocapitate ligaments, and dorsal scaphotriquetral and radiotriquetral ligaments
- Stage III: stage II plus disruption of the scapholunate and radioscapholunate ligaments with potential dorsal perilunate dislocation

In the setting of a chronic scapholunate ligament injury, arthritic changes may occur and the deformity of the capitate, lunate, and scaphoid may become static. The abnormal position of these bones can lead to wear of the articular cartilage and the surrounding articular surfaces, a condition known as scapholunate advanced collapse (SLAC).[10] As with most forms of osteoarthritis, SLAC wrist develops in stages:

- Stage I: arthritic change of the radial styloid
- Stage II: arthritic change of the scaphoid facet of the distal radius
- Stage III: arthritis of the articulation between the capitate and the lunate

The radiolunate articulation typically does not develop arthritic change in the SLAC wrist because of the normal location of the lunate within the lunate facet of the distal radius.[11]

PRESENTATION

Most patients with acute dissociative carpal instability give a history of a specific injury to the wrist, whether it is a fall on an outstretched hand, a twisting or pulling motion with immediate pain, injury from a direct blow, or some combination of

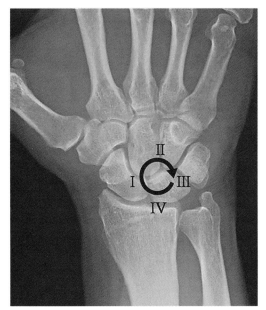

Fig. 1. Mayfield and colleagues[7] stages of progressive perilunar instability.

injuries.[12] In these cases, it is useful if the patient can recall the position of the wrist at the time of injury to determine the force vector that caused the injury. These patients typically complain of pain, swelling, or instability with lower stage injuries, progressing to an inability to use the hand with perilunate or lunate dislocations. Carpal tunnel syndrome must be evaluated, because patients with lunate dislocations have increased pressure within the carpal canal and may develop acute median nerve compression. The neurovascular status of the hand must also carefully be documented because compartment syndrome of the hand may develop.

Although acute injuries do occur, many patients present weeks to months after the initial insult, believing that they had merely sprained their wrists but without complete resolution of pain. Patients who present with subacute or chronic injuries may report pain with decreased grip strength. They may complain of weakness of the wrist, catching, clunking, or episodes of giving way. The physician must be aware of the possibility of dissociative carpal injury in even the mildest of complaints.

EXAMINATION

A patient with suspected carpal instability requires a thorough history and careful examination. The physician should palpate the wrist in an attempt to localize point tenderness. In the acute setting, swelling may make this portion of the examination difficult. It is important to determine whether the injury to the wrist is primarily radial, ulnar, or both. Pain elicited by radial or ulnar deviation of the wrist should promote suspicion of injury to the respective side of the wrist. Tenderness over the lunotriquetral or scapholunate joint indicates injury to the underlying ligament (**Figs. 2** and **3**). Pain with subjective or palpated clicking or popping may aid in diagnosis of ligamentous injury.

The Watson shift maneuver (or scaphoid shift test) was first described in 1988.[13] It is useful in determining the presence or absence of scapholunate ligament injury. In order to perform this test, the examiner sits across from the patient with a table in between. The physician grasps the radial side of the injured wrist with his same hand (eg, right hand grasps right wrist). The thumb is placed over the palmar prominence of the scaphoid while the fingers provide counterpressure on the dorsum of the wrist proximal to the carpal row. The examiner's other hand provides ulnar to radial deviation by grasping the metacarpals (**Figs. 4** and **5**). As the wrist moves beyond neutral and into radial

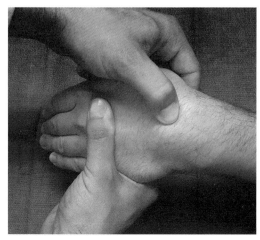

Fig. 2. Scaphoid tenderness is elicited by palpating 1 cm distal to the Lister tubercle with the wrist in slight flexion.

deviation, the dorsally directed pressure on the palmar aspect of the scaphoid may cause a subluxation. This subluxation may cause pain or apprehension in the patient, or the examiner may feel the scaphoid sublux or even dislocate out of the scaphoid fossa of the radius. The quality of wrist motion (ie, smooth or with grinding) is also noted. The pressure on the distal pole of the scaphoid is released and a clunk may be realized as the scaphoid relocates back to within the scaphoid fossa of the radius. The contralateral wrist must also be examined in order to assess for ligamentous laxity or hypermobility that may lead to a false-positive Watson shift maneuver.

An adjunctive test for scapholunate instability is the scaphoid ballottement test (**Fig. 6**).[14] The

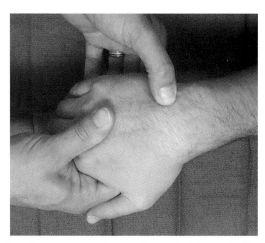

Fig. 3. Lunate tenderness is elicited by palpating 0.5 cm distal to the ulnar head with the wrist in slight flexion.

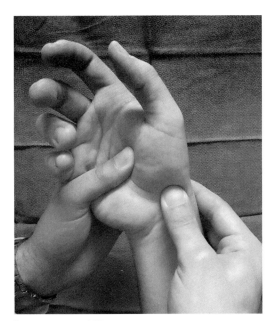

Fig. 4. Watson shift test.

patient's hand is held in pronation with fingers toward the examiner. The examiner stabilizes the lunate between the thumb dorsally and the index finger volarly. The scaphoid is stabilized in a similar manner with the examiner's opposite hand. The scaphoid is translated dorsally and volarly while observing for pain and noting the amount of translation between the scaphoid and lunate. Elicited

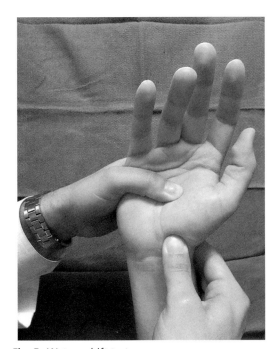

Fig. 5. Watson shift test.

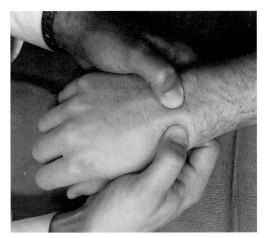

Fig. 6. Scaphoid ballottement test.

pain or increased translation compared with the contralateral side is a sign of injury to the scapholunate ligament.

Ulnar-sided wrist pain should lead to a suspicion of lunotriquetral ligament instability or injury. The Reagan test (or lunotriquetral ballottement test) is useful to identify injury to the lunotriquetral ligament.[15] The patient's hand is held in pronation with the fingers toward the examiner. The examiner stabilizes the lunate between the thumb dorsally and the index finger volarly. The triquetrum and pisiform are stabilized in a similar manner with the examiner's opposite hand. The triquetrum is translated dorsally and volarly. Elicited pain or increased translation compared with the contralateral side is a sign of injury to the lunotriquetral interosseous ligament.

The Kleinman shear test (or lunotriquetral shuck test) also indicates ligamentous injury of the ulnar wrist.[16] The patient holds the wrist in a neutral and vertical orientation with the ulnar side facing the examiner. The examiner places a thumb over the dorsum of the lunate and the index finger on the pisiform. Dorsal pressure from the examiner's index finger through the pisiform should elicit pain if there is lunotriquetral interosseous ligament injury.

STUDIES

Plain radiographs are essential when evaluating a patient for suspected carpal instability. Posteroanterior (PA), lateral, and oblique films of the wrist are obtained to evaluate static instability patterns, fractures, or dislocations. Additional radiographs should include PA films in radial and ulnar deviation, a clenched-fist or pencil view, and flexion and extension laterals to evaluate dynamic instability of the wrist. All radiographs should be performed with neutral forearm rotation.

Examination of plain films of the wrist should always include assessment of the lines of Gilula on the PA projection.[17] The 3 lines of Gilula are formed by the proximal and distal articular surfaces of the proximal row as well as the proximal articular surface of the distal row (**Fig. 7**). Any disruption of the smooth arc of these lines or overlap of the articular surfaces should prompt the examiner to search for further evidence of carpal instability.

On the PA projection, the space between the carpal bones should be uniform throughout the wrist. The width of these gaps should not change significantly with radial or ulnar deviation. Widening of the space between the scaphoid and the lunate of greater than 2 mm (the Terry-Thomas sign) may indicate injury to the scapholunate ligament (**Fig. 8**).[1] However, in dynamic scapholunate instability, the scapholunate interval may not appear widened on a normal PA view. A clenched-fist or pencil view increases the force across the wrist because of the extrinsic ligaments, loading the capitate into the proximal carpal row and producing increased widening. Contralateral wrist radiographs may be necessary to detect or determine a significant amount of widening. Ulnar and radial deviation may also aid in diagnosis of dynamic scapholunate ligament injury increasing gapping at the scapholunate or lunotriquetral joints respectively.

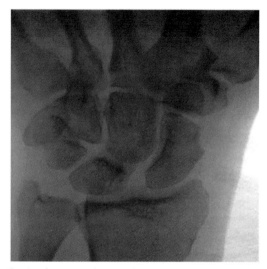

Fig. 8. The Terry-Thomas sign.

In scapholunate instability with a DISI deformity, the distal pole of the scaphoid is palmar flexed while the lunate is extended dorsally, and the cortical border of the distal pole of the scaphoid aligns with the proximal pole on standard PA imaging. The dense cortical bone forms what appears to be a ring in the scaphoid and is termed a signet-ring sign (**Fig. 9**). The lunate with increased dorsal angulation appears triangular rather than hexagonal, aiding in the diagnosis.

On the lateral projection of the normal wrist, the longitudinal axes of third metacarpal, capitate, lunate, and radius are colinear or stacked C-shaped structures (**Fig. 10**). Perilunate dislocations show colinearity of the radius and lunate while the capitate is dorsally located (**Fig. 11**). Lunate dislocations involve the dorsally, or more typical volarly,

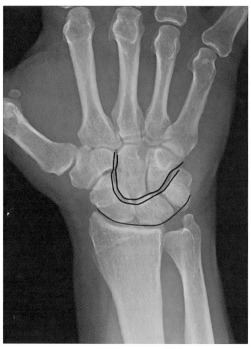

Fig. 7. The lines of Gilula.

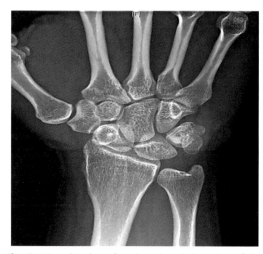

Fig. 9. PA wrist view showing signet-ring sign of the scaphoid.

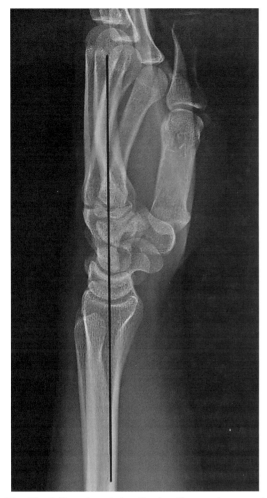

Fig. 10. Colinearity of the distal radius, capitate, and the third metacarpal.

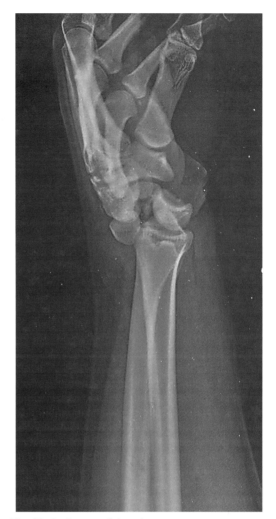

Fig. 11. Perilunate dislocation.

dislocated lunate not articulating with either the capitate or radius, and the capitate is seen to rest on the C of the distal radius.

Linscheid and colleagues[1] described the normal longitudinal axes of the scaphoid and lunate on the lateral film of the wrist. The axis of the scaphoid is a line that connects the midpoints of the proximal and distal poles. The lunate axis connects the midpoints of the convex proximal articular surface and the concave distal articular surface. The angle formed by the intersection of these axes should range from 30° to 60° (average, 47°). An angle of greater than 60° to 70° indicates potential scapholunate ligament injury and subsequent dorsiflexion of the lunate (DISI deformity), because the connecting-rod function of the scaphoid is lost (**Fig. 12**). An angle of less than 30° should promote suspicion of lunotriquetral ligament injury with volar flexion of the lunate and VISI deformity.[1]

However, a true lateral of the wrist in neutral flexion and extension must be obtained for this relationship to hold true. Flexion or extension of the wrist must be taken into account when evaluating the lateral plain film.

Magnetic resonance imaging (MRI) can be a useful adjunct study in an examination suspicious for scapholunate ligament injury when radiographs fail to confirm the diagnosis. Recent studies have shown that a 3-T MRI has sensitivity of 86% for detecting scapholunate tears and 82% for detecting lunotriquetral tears compared with arthroscopy.[18] MRI showed a specificity of 100% for both types of tears. Arthrography can also be useful in detecting a scapholunate ligament injury. Injection of gadolinium into the midcarpal joint should show the flow of dye into the midportion of the scapholunate interval, but not into the radiocarpal joint.[19]

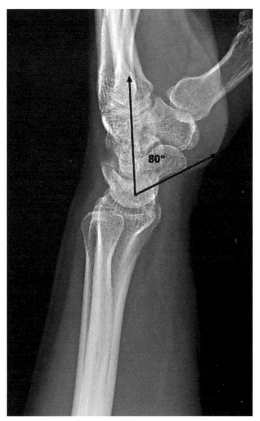

Fig. 12. Abnormal scapholunate angle of 80° representing a DISI deformity.

The gold standard for diagnosis of scapholunate or lunotriquetral ligament tears is wrist arthroscopy. Arthroscopy allows direct visualization of ligament injury, including the location and size of the insult, as well as the presence of arthritic changes within the joint space. Geissler and colleagues[20] constructed an arthroscopic classification system for intracarpal ligament tears. This 4-part scale was intended to communicate information regarding carpal alignment after intracarpal ligament tear:

- Stage I: attenuation or hemorrhage of the interosseous ligament as seen from the radiocarpal space. No incongruency of carpal alignment in the midcarpal space.
- Stage II: attenuation or hemorrhage of interosseous ligament as seen from the radiocarpal space. Incongruency or step-off of the carpal space. There may be a slight gap (less than the width of a probe) between the carpal bones.
- Stage III: incongruency or step-off of carpal alignment as seen from both the radiocarpal and midcarpal spaces. A probe may be passed through the gap between carpal bones.

- Stage IV: incongruency or step-off of carpal alignment as seen from both the radiocarpal and midcarpal spaces. There is gross instability with manipulation. A 2.7-mm arthroscope may be passed through the gap between the carpal bones (drive-through sign).

TREATMENT

Several factors must be taken into account when weighing treatment options for a patient with dissociative carpal instability. The presence of arthritis, degree of instability, the chronicity of the injury, associated injuries, and the functional demands of the patient must be considered. Patient expectations must be addressed and outcomes should be discussed with the patient before an intervention.

Dynamic scapholunate instability that presents in the acute setting may be amenable to nonoperative treatment, but the patient must understand that posttraumatic degenerative changes will likely ensue following the typical SLAC pattern. Nonsteroidal antiinflammatory drugs (NSAIDs) and activity modification are the mainstay of nonoperative treatment. Injection of corticosteroids, when used sparingly, can help to alleviate any discomfort experienced by the patient. Immobilization may reduce pain in the acutely injured wrist, followed by a course of therapy.

Surgical management of scapholunate instability depends on the acuity of the ligamentous injury, position of the scaphoid and lunate, and extent of degenerative changes, if any. The surgeon must determine partial versus complete tears, acute versus chronic tears, reducible or irreducible diastasis, and the presence or absence of degenerative tears. This identification guides the surgeon toward treatment (**Fig. 13**).

PARTIAL SCAPHOLUNATE LIGAMENT TEARS/ DYNAMIC INSTABILITY WITHOUT DIASTASIS

For those patients with dynamic instability and partial scapholunate tears, arthroscopic debridement has yielded positive results.[21] However simple debridement alone for complete scapholunate tears is unsatisfactory.[22] Instability of the scapholunate ligament may be treated with aggressive arthroscopic debridement and percutaneous pinning with Kirschner wires (K-wires). Pins placed dorsally into the scaphoid and the lunate are used as joysticks to reduce the joint. Once proper alignment is restored, the scaphoid and lunate are pinned in place for a period of up to 10 weeks. Cast immobilization may be used to protect the construct. Although the results of this procedure

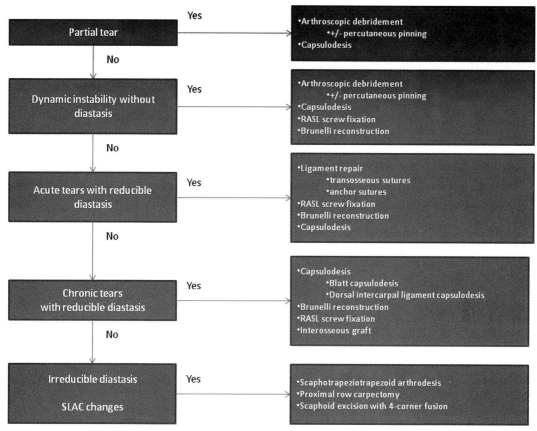

Fig. 13. Treatment algorithm for scapholunate ligament injury. RASL, reduction and association of the scaphoid and lunate.

have also proved suboptimal, they remain an option for patients reluctant to undergo open treatment or reconstruction.[23]

ACUTE, REDUCIBLE SCAPHOLUNATE LIGAMENT TEARS

Acute but reducible scapholunate diastasis is treated with an open reduction of the scapholunate joint and repair of the ligament. A dorsal approach allows repair of the stout dorsal subregion of the ligament and also provides the option of adding a dorsal capsulodesis.[24] The scapholunate ligament is typically torn from the scaphoid and remains attached the lunate. Drill holes are created in the proximal pole of the scaphoid that exit at the origin of the scapholunate ligament. Sutures are passed through these holes and function to reapproximate the ligament to the scaphoid. Suture anchors placed at the origin of the scapholunate ligament may be substitute for transosseous holes. K-wires may be used as joysticks to help effectuate the reduction. Also the scaphoid and lunate may be transfixed with K-wires to protect the repair.

If repair of the scapholunate ligament is not possible, a headless compression screw may be used to approximate the scapholunate ligament via an open or arthroscopic approach called a reduction and association of the scaphoid and lunate (RASL) procedure. After reduction of the scapholunate interval, the screw is placed from radius to ulnar into the scaphoid and lunate bones. The screw is used to approximate the scapholunate interval and provide stability. As the wrist undergoes motion, the scapholunate interval rotates around the centrally nonthreaded portion of the screw. Arthroscopic RASL screw fixation controls pain and improves wrist function while preserving wrist range of motion.[25]

CHRONIC, REDUCIBLE SCAPHOLUNATE LIGAMENT TEARS

Chronic, reducible scapholunate diastasis is treated according to the viability of the scapholunate ligament and the presence or absence of degeneration. The ligament is more likely to be scarred down and irreparable in the setting of a chronic tear; however, if the ligament remains viable, repair may be attempted as discussed earlier. Irreparable ligament tears without extensive osteochondral degeneration may be treated with scapholunate ligament reconstruction. Capsulodesis and tendon weaves are reconstruction techniques that provide adequate stabilization while minimizing loss of volar flexion. RASL cannulated screw fixation is indicated for irreparable scapholunate ligament damage. Bone-tissue-bone autograft is an alternative treatment that can be technically demanding.[26]

The Blatt capsulodesis technique tethers the scaphoid to the distal radius via a flap of dorsal capsuloligamentous tissue secured with suture anchors; however, this can cause a loss of wrist flexion.[27] More recently, a modification of this technique has been used that tethers the scaphoid to the triquetrum, decreasing the loss of wrist flexion that can be seen with the former procedure.[28] This so-called dorsal intercarpal ligament capsulodesis leads to acceptable long-term function of the wrist, at the cost of early arthritic degeneration.[29]

The Brunelli technique stabilizes the scaphoid in a reduced position by passing the flexor carpi radialis tendon through an interosseous scaphoid tunnel and onto the distal radius (**Figs. 14** and **15**).[30] Garcia and colleagues[31] recently modified this technique to pass the tendon through the scaphoid, weave it through the dorsal radiotriquetral ligament,

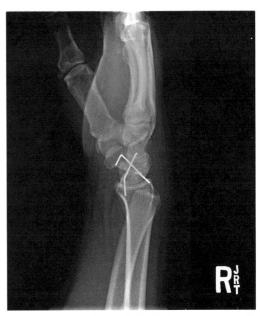

Fig. 15. Lateral radiograph depicting a postoperative Brunelli reconstruction reinforced by percutaneous K-wires.

and then terminally attach the ligament to the lunate. This technique is referred to as the triligament tenodesis because it is designed to stabilize the scaphotrapeziotrapezoidal, scapholunate, and dorsal radiotriquetral ligaments while minimizing the loss of volar flexion that accompanies a traditional Brunelli technique.

Although originally described for Geissler type III degeneration, RASL screw fixation has been used for a growing number of indications. As mentioned earlier, headless compression screw fixation is a recognized treatment of acute but irreparable scapholunate tears. Chronic tears with a reducible scapholunate interval are amenable to this treatment as well. Arthroscopic RASL fixation has good results that rival those of soft tissue procedures such as the Blatt or Brunelli.[25]

Bone-tissue-bone autograft has been proposed as treatment of chronic, reducible scapholunate ligament injury.[26] Donor sites include the navicular-medial cuneiform, bone–extensor retinaculum–bone from the distal radius, bone-ligament-bone from the second and third metacarpal base, and bone-ligament-bone from the capitate and hamate. After reduction of the scapholunate interval, a trough is made within the dorsal scaphoid and lunate bones. The bone-ligament-bone autograft is fitted within this trough and secured with small 1.1-mm or 1.3-mm screws. Although long-term data are lacking on these procedures, results have been promising to date.[26]

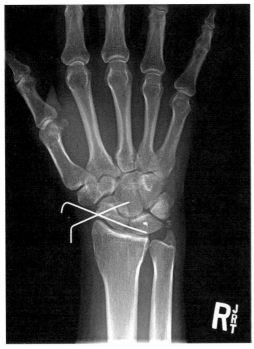

Fig. 14. PA radiograph of a postoperative Brunelli reconstruction reinforced by percutaneous K-wires.

IRREDUCIBLE DIASTASIS/DEGENERATIVE CHANGES (SLAC WRIST)

Symptomatic patients with irreducible injuries, or those who fail scapholunate ligament repair, can be treated with several salvage techniques. Scaphotrapeziotrapezoid (or triscaphe) arthrodesis was first described in 1967 and can produce successful long-term results.[32] Proximal row carpectomy may be performed if the proximal pole of the capitate does not show significant arthritic change; however, long-term satisfaction is limited, and thus a proximal row carpectomy is typically reserved for patients more than 35 years of age.[33] Scaphoid excision with fusion of the capitate, hamate, lunate, and triquetrum shows equivocal results compared with proximal row carpectomy for SLAC wrists at 19 months and is the procedure of choice in a young or high-demand patient.[34]

Isolated lunotriquetral ligament injuries are less common than scapholunate ligament injuries and are treated differently. In most cases of acute and chronic lunotriquetral instability, conservative management is the first line of therapy. NSAIDs, activity modification, and corticosteroid injections combined with wrist immobilization are used.[6]

Acute or chronic lunotriquetral injuries that show a VISI deformity or fail conservative treatment can be addressed operatively. The goal of treatment should be a reestablishment of the lunocapitate axis. In the acute setting, an attempt can be made to repair the lunotriquetral ligament. Similar to scapholunate ligament repair, bone tunnels and suture anchors can be used to provide a stable construct.[12]

Chronic lunotriquetral instability should be treated with either ligament reconstruction or arthrodesis. Reconstruction of the ligament with extensor carpi ulnaris tendon has yielded good results at the 5-year mark.[12] Recent studies have shown that arthrodesis of the lunotriquetral joint with autologous bone graft secured by either K-wire, Herbert screw, or Arbeitsgemeinschaft für Osteosynthesefragen compression screw is complicated by nonunion, impingement, and RSD.[12,35,36] Ligament reconstruction has shown the most promising results, with fewer complications and less need for reoperation than either repair of the ligament or arthrodesis of the joint.[12]

SUMMARY

The scaphoid serves as the connecting rod between the proximal and dorsal carpal rows and is stabilized by the scapholunate ligament (directly) and lunotriquetral ligament (indirectly). Disruption of either of these ligaments leads to a pattern of instability that, left untreated, leads to altered mechanics of the wrist and ultimately debilitating arthritis and collapse. Although arthroscopy remains the gold standard for diagnosis of these injuries, plain films and arthrograms are useful adjuncts. In the acute setting, conservative treatment may be attempted, but recalcitrant cases require surgical stabilization. Salvage procedures are also available for those patients who fail initial stabilization. Dissociative carpal instability remains a challenging problem, but successful treatment can be rewarding for both the patient and the surgeon.

REFERENCES

1. Linscheid RL, Dobyns JH, Beabout JW, et al. Traumatic instability of the wrist. Diagnosis, classification, and pathomechanics. J Bone Joint Surg Am 1972;54: 1612–32.
2. Berger RA. The gross and histologic anatomy of the scapholunate interosseous ligament. J Hand Surg 1996;21:170–8.
3. Katz DA, Green JK, Werner FW, et al. Capsuloligamentous restraints to dorsal and palmar carpal translation. J Hand Surg 2003;28:610–3.
4. Kitay A, Wolfe SW. Scapholunate instability: current concepts in diagnosis and management. J Hand Surg 2012;37:2175–96.
5. Kuo CE, Wolfe SW. Scapholunate instability: current concepts in diagnosis and management. J Hand Surg 2008;33:998–1013.
6. Shin AY, Battaglia MJ, Bishop AT. Lunotriquetral instability: diagnosis and treatment. J Am Acad Orthop Surg 2000;8:170–9.
7. Mayfield JK, Johnson RP, Kilcoyne RK. Carpal dislocations: pathomechanics and progressive perilunar instability. J Hand Surg 1980;5:226–41.
8. Richards RS, Bennett JD, Roth JH, et al. Arthroscopic diagnosis of intra-articular soft tissue injuries associated with distal radial fractures. J Hand Surg 1997;22:772–6.
9. Murray PM, Palmer CG, Shin AY. The mechanism of ulnar-sided perilunate instability of the wrist: a cadaveric study and 6 clinical cases. J Hand Surg 2012;37:721–8.
10. Watson HK, Ballet FL. The SLAC wrist: scapholunate advanced collapse pattern of degenerative arthritis. J Hand Surg 1984;9:358–65.
11. Ashmead D, Watson HK, Damon C, et al. Scapholunate advanced collapse wrist salvage. J Hand Surg 1994;19:741–50.
12. Shin AY, Weinstein LP, Berger RA, et al. Treatment of isolated injuries of the lunotriquetral ligament. A comparison of arthrodesis, ligament reconstruction and ligament repair. J Bone Joint Surg Br 2001;83: 1023–8.

13. Watson HK, Ashmead D, Makhlouf MV. Examination of the scaphoid. J Hand Surg 1988;13:657–60.

14. Green DP. Green's operative hand surgery. 5th edition. Philadelphia: Elsevier/Churchill Livingstone; 2005.

15. Reagan DS, Linscheid RL, Dobyns JH. Lunotriquetral sprains. J Hand Surg 1984;9:502–14.

16. Sachar K. Ulnar-sided wrist pain: evaluation and treatment of triangular fibrocartilage complex tears, ulnocarpal impaction syndrome, and lunotriquetral ligament tears. J Hand Surg 2012;37:1489–500.

17. Gilula LA. Carpal injuries: analytic approach and case exercises. AJR Am J Roentgenol 1979;133: 503–17.

18. Magee T. Comparison of 3-T MRI and arthroscopy of intrinsic wrist ligament and TFCC tears. AJR Am J Roentgenol 2009;192:80–5.

19. Tirman RM, Weber ER, Snyder LL, et al. Midcarpal wrist arthrography for detection of tears of the scapholunate and lunotriquetral ligaments. AJR Am J Roentgenol 1985;144:107–8.

20. Geissler WB, Freeland AE, Savoie FH, et al. Intracarpal soft-tissue lesions associated with an intra-articular fracture of the distal end of the radius. J Bone Joint Surg Am 1996;78:357–65.

21. Ruch DS, Poehling GG. Arthroscopic management of partial scapholunate and lunotriquetral injuries of the wrist. J Hand Surg 1996;21:412–7.

22. Weiss AP, Sachar K, Glowacki KA. Arthroscopic debridement alone for intercarpal ligament tears. J Hand Surg 1997;22:344–9.

23. Darlis NA, Kaufmann RA, Giannoulis F, et al. Arthroscopic debridement and closed pinning for chronic dynamic scapholunate instability. J Hand Surg 2006; 31:418–24.

24. Lavernia CJ, Cohen MS, Taleisnik J. Treatment of scapholunate dissociation by ligamentous repair and capsulodesis. J Hand Surg 1992;17:354–9.

25. Caloia M, Caloia H, Pereira E. Arthroscopic scapholunate joint reduction. Is an effective treatment for irreparable scapholunate ligament tears? Clin Orthop Relat Res 2012;470:972–8.

26. Harvey EJ, Berger RA, Osterman AL, et al. Bone-tissue-bone repairs for scapholunate dissociation. J Hand Surg 2007;32:256–64.

27. Wintman BI, Gelberman RH, Katz JN. Dynamic scapholunate instability: results of operative treatment with dorsal capsulodesis. J Hand Surg 1995;20: 971–9.

28. Szabo RM, Slater RR Jr, Palumbo CF, et al. Dorsal intercarpal ligament capsulodesis for chronic, static scapholunate dissociation: clinical results. J Hand Surg 2002;27:978–84.

29. Megerle K, Bertel D, Germann G, et al. Long-term results of dorsal intercarpal ligament capsulodesis for the treatment of chronic scapholunate instability. J Bone Joint Surg Br 2012;94:1660–5.

30. Brunelli GA, Brunelli GR. A new surgical technique for carpal instability with scapholunate dissociation. Surg Technol Int 1996;5:370–4.

31. Garcia-Elias M, Lluch AL, Stanley JK. Three-ligament tenodesis for the treatment of scapholunate dissociation: indications and surgical technique. J Hand Surg 2006;31:125–34.

32. Kleinman WB. Long-term study of chronic scapholunate instability treated by scapho-trapezio-trapezoid arthrodesis. J Hand Surg 1989;14:429–45.

33. Ali MH, Rizzo M, Shin AY, et al. Long-term outcomes of proximal row carpectomy: a minimum of 15-year follow-up. Hand (N Y) 2012;7:72–8.

34. Cohen MS, Kozin SH. Degenerative arthritis of the wrist: proximal row carpectomy versus scaphoid excision and four-corner arthrodesis. J Hand Surg 2001;26:94–104.

35. McAuliffe JA, Dell PC, Jaffe R. Complications of intercarpal arthrodesis. J Hand Surg 1993;18:1121–8.

36. Vandesande W, De Smet L, Van Ransbeeck H. Lunotriquetral arthrodesis, a procedure with a high failure rate. Acta Orthop Belg 2001;67:361–7.

Kienböck Disease

Danielle Cross, MD[a], Kristofer S. Matullo, MD[b],*

KEYWORDS

- Kienböck disease • Lunate osteonecrosis • Lunate AVN • Avascular necrosis • Lunate • Kienböck

KEY POINTS

- Kienböck disease is defined by avascular necrosis of the lunate with a predictable pattern of lunate collapse, carpal change, and degeneration, resulting from an apparent combination of vascular, anatomic, and traumatic insults.
- Advancements are still being made with regards to the cause, pathophysiology, and preferred method of treatment of each of the various stages of Kienböck disease.
- Although the goals of pain relief, motion preservation, strength maintenance, and function outcomes are paramount to success, there is no 1 procedure that consistently and reliably achieves these outcomes.
- With further advancements in treatment and results of long-term outcome studies, answers should be obtained to some of these still unresolved topics.

INTRODUCTION

Kienböck disease, also known as avascular necrosis (AVN) or osteomalacia of the lunate, was first described in 1843 by Peste[1] through his cadaveric work and observations of lunate collapse. However, the term Kienböck disease was coined after Dr Robert Kienböck, an Austrian radiologist, when he presented clinical and radiographic evidence of 16 patients with osteomalacia of the lunate in 1910.[2] He described a stepwise progression of disease from isolated proximal lunate involvement, to fragmentation and collapse of the lunate, evolving to radiocarpal involvement with degenerative changes. He believed the osteomalacia to be a result of "a disturbance in the nutrition of the lunate caused by rupture of the ligaments and blood vessels during contusions, sprains, or subluxations.[2]"

Since the early descriptions by Kienböck, there has been research to explore the cause, pathophysiology, staging, treatments, and outcomes of Kienböck disease.

CAUSE AND PATHOPHYSIOLOGY

The cause of Kienböck disease is still debated, but it is likely multifactorial and seems to result from varying degrees of anatomic factors, interrupted vascularity, and traumatic insults to the lunate.

Various anatomic and mechanical factors have been associated with the development of Kienböck disease. Hulten[3] was the first to describe the relationship between Kienböck disease and ulnar negative variance. In 1928, he described a series of patients with Kienböck disease, in whom 78% of affected patients were noted to have ulnar negative variance, and 23% of individuals with neutral or positive ulnar variance were affected. His work was followed by Gelberman and colleagues,[4] who also found a significant relationship between ulnar negativity and Kienböck disease when they studied various anatomic and vascular differences among 35 cadaver specimens.

Antuna Zapico[5] described 3 types of lunate morphologies and related them to ulnar variance

The authors have nothing to disclose.
[a] Department of Orthopaedic Surgery, St. Luke's University Hospital, 801 Ostrum Street, Bethlehem, PA 18015, USA; [b] Division of Hand Surgery, Department of Orthopaedic Surgery, St. Luke's University Hospital and Health Network, PPH-2, 801 Ostrum Street, Bethlehem, PA 18015, USA
* Corresponding author.
E-mail address: Kristofer.Matullo@sluhn.org

Orthop Clin N Am 45 (2014) 141–152
http://dx.doi.org/10.1016/j.ocl.2013.09.004
0030-5898/14/$ – see front matter © 2014 Elsevier Inc. All rights reserved.

and described their association with Kienböck disease. A type I lunate has a proximal apex, which is more likely to be seen in wrists with ulnar negative variance. In type II and III lunates, the shape is more rectangular and is associated with ulnar neutral or positive wrists. Type I lunates were associated with higher rates of stress and fragmentation under loading, and the investigators concluded that they were the weakest configuration. Despite this evidence, several subsequent studies have failed to show a definitive relationship between ulnar variance and Kienböck disease.[6–8]

Other studies have described the relationship between a lower angle of radial inclination and Kienböck disease.[8,9] Although there is no general consensus regarding radiocarpal anatomy and the development of Kienböck disease, there seems to be a relationship between unequal load distribution through the radiocarpal joint, whereby the lunate receives an abnormal distribution of the force, and the lunate subsequently becomes at risk for the development of Kienböck disease.

The vascular supply to the lunate is variable, but most have both a dorsal and volar nutritional supply.[4] Three major patterns of vascularity have been described: Y, X, and I types, which refer to the geometric branching of the intraosseous arteries.[4] In the I pattern, there is a single vessel supplying the lunate, which may increase the risk for the development of osteonecrosis. It has been reported that approximately 7% to 23% of patients have a single contributing vessel to the lunate,[4,10] and up to 31% of individuals have minimal branching of the anastamotic vessels that provide nutrition to the lunate.[10] In addition, AVN of the lunate has been linked to a vascular insult caused by fracture, ligament collapse, primary circulatory collapse, systemic disease, ligamentous collapse, and venous congestion.[11–15] However, none of these occurs with significant regularity to allow for generalized screening.[11,12] Schiltenwolf and colleagues[16] concluded that necrotic lunates showed significantly higher levels of intraosseous vascular congestion compared with normal lunates, but it was unclear whether or not this was related to lunate collapse or was a cause of the disease process itself.

The relationship between Kienböck disease and traumatic insults has been studied extensively, and there seems to be a link between trauma and the development of osteonecrosis in the lunate. Repetitive microtrauma, such as that seen in heavy laborers, seems to play a role, but there is often no association between a single traumatic event and the development of Kienböck disease.[17] Although early increased radiodensity of the lunate can be seen after a perilunate dislocation, the collapse and fragmentation that are seen in Kienböck disease rarely occur in this subset of patients, as confirmed by Takami and colleagues.[18] The volar lunate vasculature typically remains attached to the volar capsule during this injury, thus preserving the blood supply of the lunate.[13]

Although there is no single definitive cause of Kienböck disease, a complex interplay of vascular and anatomic variations, combined with varying degrees of microtrauma and insults, contribute to its development.

CLINICAL PRESENTATION

Kienböck disease most commonly affects men between the ages of 20 and 40 years.[11] Many patients describe a history of trauma, but this is not always present. Although symptoms can vary depending on their stage at initial presentation, patients typically present with pain localized to the radiolunate facet, decreased motion, swelling, and weakness in the affected hand. Pain is classically insidious in onset, often related to activity, and can be present for extended periods before presentation. The disease is rarely bilateral.

Physical examination reveals tenderness over the dorsal lunate and radiolunate facet. An effusion or bogginess overlying the radiocarpal joint is not an uncommon finding. Motion in the flexion and extension arc is often decreased, and average grip strength may decrease up to 50% of the contralateral side.[19]

RADIOGRAPHIC IMAGING

Standard neutral rotation posteroanterior (PA) and lateral radiographs of the affected hand should be ordered on any patient suspected to have Kienböck disease. Plain radiographs may be negative early in the disease process, but typically progress to show increased lunate density, which indicates osteonecrosis. With worsening disease, collapse of the lunate and fragmentation of the lunate are visualized. Advanced disease yields proximal migration of the capitate, dorsal intercalary segmental instability (DISI), showing scaphoid flexion coupled with lunate extension and degenerative disease involving the radiocarpal joint.

Advanced imaging can aid in the diagnosis and staging of Kienböck disease. Bone scintigraphy, which has largely been replaced by the ease and convenience of magnetic resonance imaging (MRI), can detect early stages of the disease with increased signal uptake. MRI typically shows decreased signal intensity on T1-weighted and T2-weighted images indicating impaired vascularity. In patients with other diseases, such as perilunate dislocation or ulnar impaction syndrome, changes within the lunate may appear similar to the osteonecrotic changes seen in Kienböck disease. However, these changes are often focal and nonprogressive, which is different from the uniform osteonecrotic changes seen in the lunate of patients with Kienböck disease. Hashizume and colleagues[20] compared diagnostic modalities and concluded that although MRI is useful in detecting early stages of disease before collapse has occurred, other imaging modalities such as computed tomography (CT) or tomography best characterize lunate necrosis and trabecular destruction once collapse has occurred.

Trispiral tomography is another useful adjunct to the diagnosis of Kienböck disease. In a study conducted by Quezner and colleagues,[21] 105 patients with radiographic evidence of stage I disease were evaluated with trispiral tomography, 87% of patients were upgraded to stage II after imaging. Likewise 71% of patients with stage II disease and 9% of patients with stage III disease were upgraded to stage III and IV, respectively, after trispiral tomography imaging. However, this imaging modality is not widely available.

STAGING

Stahl[22] originally described the classification of Kienböck disease in 1947. Lichtman and colleagues[11] introduced a modified classification scheme that has remained the most frequently used. A summary of the Lichtman classification can be found in **Table 1**.

Table 1
Summary of Lichtman classification of Kienböck disease

Stage I	Normal radiographs, ± linear fracture lines. MRI shows uniform signal decrease on T1-weighted images. Bone scan positive but nonspecific
Stage II	Plain radiographs show lunate sclerosis, ± fracture lines. No collapse of lunate
Stage IIIA	Lunate collapse, with maintenance of carpal height and alignment
Stage IIIB	Lunate collapse plus any of the following: loss of carpal height, proximal capitate migration, flexed and rotated scaphoid
Stage IV	Stage IIIB + radiocarpal or midcarpal degenerative changes

Stage I

Patients presenting with stage I disease typically complain of nonspecific, intermittent wrist pain and synovitis, which mimic a wrist sprain. Plain films are either normal or show small linear compression fractures through the lunate. There is no collapse, sclerosis, or increased radiodensity of the lunate.

MRI shows uniformly decreased signal uptake on both T1-weighted and T2-weighted images, indicating osteonecrosis of the lunate. If revascularization is occurring, such as after operative intervention, increased signal uptake on the T2-weighted images would be noted.

Bone scintigraphy at this stage typically shows decreased signal uptake and changes related to reactive synovitis.

Stage II

Stage II is characterized clinically by increased swelling, varying degrees of stiffness, and progressive pain. Radiographs show lunate sclerosis, with or without compression fracture lines. The lunate appears more radiodense, but there is no evidence of collapse and lunate height is maintained. The remainder of the carpus remains without degenerative change and the relationship between the lunate and the proximal carpal row is maintained.

Although other pathologic conditions may create increased sclerosis of the lunate, such as after a perilunate dislocation or with ulnar impaction syndrome, this process is typically focal and generally without significant progression. Patients with Kienböck disease present with diffuse lunate changes that are typically progressive. Ulnar variance (negative, neutral, or positive) should be noted.

Fig. 1 shows an individual with stage II disease.

Stage III

Stage III disease is defined by continued sclerosis and collapse of the lunate. This stage is divided into 2 separate subgroups, depending on the alignment and maintenance of carpal relationships. Attention must be paid to the scapholunate angle to evaluate for a DISI deformity as well as the carpal height. Carpal height is measured as the distance between the distal articular surface of the capitate to the lunate fossa of the distal radius. The carpal height ration is the carpal height divided by the length of the third metacarpal and is approximately 0.53.[23] A decrease of the carpal height and carpal height ratio suggests collapse or osteoarthritic change within the carpus.

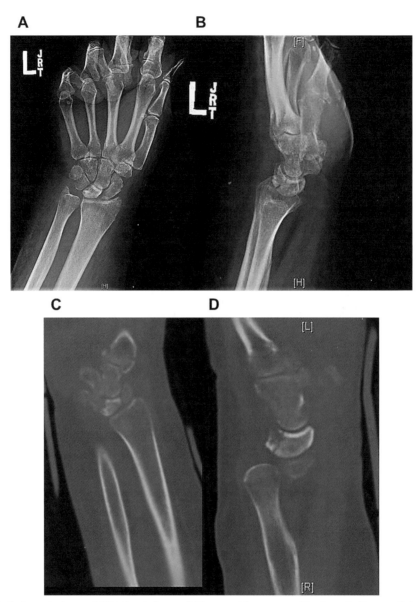

Fig. 1. (*A*) Anteriposterior and (*B*) lateral views of 66-year-old woman with stage II disease. Note the sclerosis and fracturing of the lunate, but lack of collapse. (*C*) and (*D*) show anteriposterior and lateral CT images of the same individual, which again emphasize the extent of lunate sclerosis and fracture, but no lunate or carpal collapse.

Stage IIIA is characterized by collapse of the lunate, with preservation of carpal height and intercarpal alignment. Thus, the capitate has not migrated proximally and the scaphoid has not assumed a flexed position. On a lateral radiograph, the lunate appears widened in the anteroposterior plane as a result of the coronal plane collapse. The scapholunate angle is also preserved at –10° to 10°.

Stage IIIB is characterized by both collapse of the lunate and characteristic changes of the surrounding capitate and scaphoid. The capitate migrates proximally, and carpal height becomes diminished. As the scaphoid flexes and subsequently rotates, a DISI pattern may become evident. Scaphoid flexion may be appreciated on a PA radiograph as a cortical ring sign.[13] The triquetrium shifts ulnarly as a result of the surrounding carpal changes and widening at the scapholunate interval.

Symptoms at this stage have typically progressed from vague wrist pain and synovitis to symptoms of instability, clunking with radial and ulnar deviation, progressive pain, and decreased grip strength. An example of stage IIIB disease is shown in **Fig. 2**.

Stage IV

Stage IV disease is characterized by progressive carpal collapse, leading to radiocarpal and midcarpal degenerative changes. Radiographs show classic joint space narrowing, subchondral sclerosis, degenerative cysts, and osteophyte formation. Symptoms have typically progressed to stiffness, constant pain, and swelling.

TREATMENT

There are several treatment options for Kienböck disease, largely based on the stage at presentation. Although options vary, they typically fall into several broad categories: unload the lunate, revascularize the lunate, or treat carpal instability and

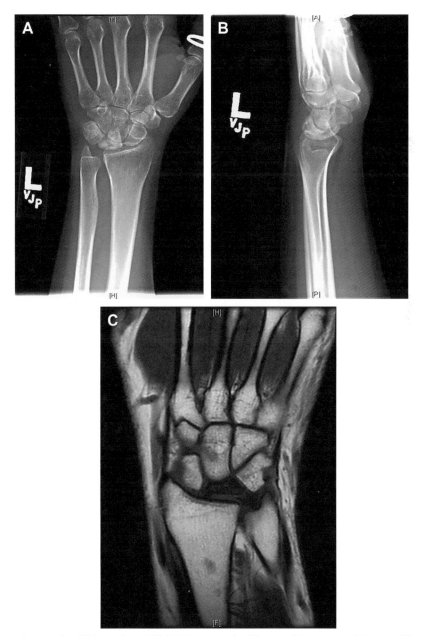

Fig. 2. (*A*) Anterioposterior (*B*) lateral and (*C*) MRI images of a 23-year-old woman with stage IIIB disease. Note the amount of fragmentation, collapse, and loss of carpal height.

collapse with salvage procedures. A summary is given in **Table 2**.

Stage I

Conservative treatment with 3 months of immobilization is typically recommended first for patients with stage I disease, although some have argued that this has minimal effect.[22,24] Taniguchi and colleagues[25] reported 35-year outcomes on a series of 20 patients, and found that although 70% of patients had radiographic progression of the disease, only 20% were symptomatic. Likewise, Kristensen and colleagues[26] followed 46 patients treated nonoperatively for a minimum of 5 years, and reported that 66% of patients had arthritic changes on imaging but only 25% were symptomatic. Delaere and colleagues[27] followed 21 surgically treated patients and 22 conservatively treated patients for 65 months and found no difference in outcomes, but did find change in social activities and loss of motion in nearly 25% of the operative group.

However, in contrast to these findings, several studies have reported poor outcomes with nonoperative management of stage I disease. Keith and colleagues[28] reported decreased DASH (Disabilities of the Arm, Shoulder and Hand) scores, motion, and grip strength in a series of 33 patients treated nonoperatively. Likewise, Lichtman[11] reported results of 22 patients treated nonoperatively, and results were poor: 17 patients had disease progression, and 5 patients had no improvement in symptoms.

Thus, although a 3-month trial of immobilization for stage I disease should be considered, the patients should continue to be monitored and if symptoms or radiographs progress, surgical discussion should commence.

Stage II or IIIA with Negative Ulnar Variance

Stage II and IIIA are considered together when considering treatment options. Although lunate collapse has occurred with stage IIIA, there remains a normal intercarpal relationship. Decreased vascularity has occurred with both stages.

The goal of treatment of stage II and IIIA with ulnar negative variance is generally centered toward unloading the lunate in an attempt to reduce intracarpal stress and allow for revascularization. Radial shortening osteotomies or ulnar lengthening procedures are joint leveling procedures that redistribute lunate load forces. The desired outcome is ulnar neutrality to 1 mm of ulnar positivity.[13] Greater ulnar positive variance may result in ulnar impaction against the lunate or triquetrium, and cause ulnar-sided wrist pain or disease.

Horii and colleagues[29] developed a two-dimensional model that looked at various joint leveling procedures in an attempt to quantify the amount of lunate unloading. Either ulnar lengthening or radial shortening of 4 mm led to a 45% decrease in force across the radiolunate joint. Likewise, Trumble and colleagues[30] investigated treatment of Kienböck disease and reported that a 70% decrease in lunate strain was seen with ulnar lengthening, radial shortening, and scaphotrapeziotrapezoidal (STT) fusion. Specific to radial shortening and ulnar lengthening procedures, these investigators noted that 90% of the reduction in lunate strain occurred with the first 2 mm of length change. Joint leveling procedures were preferred for this stage of disease, because it maintained wrist motion, whereas STT fusion resulted in decreased radial deviation and wrist extension. Nakamura and colleagues[31] concluded that radial shortening greater than 4 mm led to ulnar-sided wrist pain, and thus, 3 mm should be the maximum amount of radial shortening attempted.

Radial shortening

With regards to clinical outcomes of joint leveling procedures, Quenzer and colleagues[32] reported results on 68 patients who underwent a radial

Table 2 Treatment of Kienböck disease	
Stage I	Cast immobilization for 3 mo. If disease progresses after 3 mo, consider stage II/IIIA treatment options
Stage II/IIIA with ulnar negativity	Joint leveling procedures; radial shortening osteotomy, ulnar lengthening osteotomy
Stage II/IIIA with ulnar positivity or neutrality	Revascularization procedures ± stabilization; capitate shortening; radial wedge or dome osteotomies; core decompression; combination of revascularization with joint leveling procedures
Stage IIIB	PRC, radial shortening osteotomy, limited intercarpal arthrodesis (STT or SC fusion), lunate excision with interposition grafting
Stage IV	PRC, wrist arthrodesis, wrist arthroplasty, wrist denervation

shortening osteotomy; a 93% decrease in pain was reported at an average follow-up of 52 months. Grip strength increased in 74% of patients, whereas motion improved in 52% of patients and decreased in 19% of patients. In addition, one-third of patients showed signs of revascularization. Watanabe and colleagues[33] reported long-term outcomes of radial shortening osteotomy procedures for stage II and IIIA disease, with an average 21-year follow-up, and found that motion and grip strength remained greater than 80% compared with the contralateral wrist, average DASH scores were 8, and patient satisfaction was high. Other studies looking at long-term outcomes of joint leveling procedures have concluded that radial shortening osteotomy is an effective, safe, and reliable procedure for stage II and IIIA disease.[34] Radial shortening osteotomies should not be considered for patients who have progressed to stage IIIB disease, because the results are often less favorable.[33,34]

Ulnar shortening

As an alternative to radial shortening, ulnar lengthening procedures achieve the same goal of unloading the lunate to allow for revascularization. Linscheid described an ulnar lengthening technique using an iliac crest bone graft. He reported results of 64 patients over a 14-year period and described high patient satisfaction, favorable range of motion, and improved grip strength. However, there was a 22% complication rate, which included 9 patients with a nonunion and 5 patients with ulnar impingement syndrome. Seven patients required an additional procedure.[35] Although this surgery is an option for patients with stage II and IIIA disease, more favorable results with less morbidity and fewer complications are typically seen with radial shortening procedures.

Stage II and IIIA with Ulnar Neutral or Positive Variance

Direct revascularization allows the potential for salvage of the lunate and possible reversal of destruction of the lunate through neoangiogenesis. Many revascularization procedures have been described, including distal radius pedicle grafts, vascularized pisiform grafts, fourth or fifth extensor compartment artery transfers, or first, second, or third dorsal metacarpal artery transfers.[36–38] Sheetz and colleagues[36] reported the anatomic relationships of several vascularized pedicles from the distal radius and ulna that can be harvested and transferred to the lunate for revascularization.

Revascularization

Hori and colleagues[39] described results of a vascularization procedure that transferred the second dorsal metacarpal vascular pedicle to the lunate.[38] Long-term outcomes of this procedure included reduced pain in 50 of 51 patients and improved strength in all 51 patients. Despite these favorable outcomes, 10% showed progression of lunate fragmentation, and 20% showed increased degenerative changes. Bochud and colleagues[37] reported 2-year outcomes of 32 patients treated with a vascularized pisiform transfer and found that 95% of patients showed restoration of lunate anatomy, but only 33% of patients maintained this correction. Fair to poor results were seen in nearly half of cases at final follow-up. Alternatively, Moran and colleagues[40,41] described revascularization in 48 patients with an average 10-year follow-up. Significant pain relief was related by 98% of patients, and MRI evidence of lunate revascularization occurred in 60% of patients.

Osteotomies

Osteotomies provide an alternative to revascularization and include capitate shortening osteotomies with or without capitohamate fusion, radial closing-wedge osteotomies, and radial-dome osteotomies.[7,9,42] The goal of these various procedures is to unload the lunate in an attempt to decrease stress across the radiolunate joint, to allow for revascularization and prevention of disease progression. Almquist described a capitate shortening procedure and its associated results, reporting 83% revascularization of the lunate.[42] In addition to this, Viola and colleagues[43] reported significant reduction in load across the radiolunate joint after capitate shortening osteotomy with capitohamate fusion. Radial closing-wedge osteotomies have been described for patients with ulnar positive wrists and act to reduce radial inclination and, subsequently, the stress across the radiolunate articulation.[9,44] Various long-term studies have reported favorable outcomes in terms of pain, grip strength, and motion, despite evidence of disease progression.[33,44,45] Takahara and colleagues[46] recently described the surgical technique of radial closing-wedge shortening osteotomy for patients with ulnar positive wrists, and recommend 5° to 10° of a closing wedge with a total of 2 mm of shortening.

Core decompression

Core decompression of the radius and ulna creates a local vascular healing response and has been suggested for patients with stage I to IIIA disease. Illarramendi and colleagues[47] described 10-year follow-up results of 22 patients treated with distal radial and ulna metaphyseal core decompression, using cortical windows and a small curette. Average grip strength was 75%, and motion was 77% compared with the contralateral wrist. Seventy-three percent of patients reported no pain, and 20 patients were able to return to their occupations.

Stage IIIB

By this stage, the surrounding carpus has been altered because of progressive lunate collapse and fragmentation, with resulting scaphoid flexion, proximal capitate migration, and decreased carpal height. Thus, procedures are needed to address the destabilized carpus, prevent further carpal collapse, and decrease load across the radiolunate joint. There are several procedures that can accomplish these goals, including proximal row carpectomy (PRC); STT and scaphocapitate (SC) arthrodesis; radial shortening osteotomy; fusion with or without lunate excision; and interposition grafting.

PRC

PRC is a procedure that excises the scaphoid, lunate, and triquetrium, transferring load from the capitate directly to the lunate facet of the distal radius. Wall and Stern[48] recently reviewed PRC as a treatment option for advanced Kienböck disease and reported favorable results, few complications, painless motion, and adequate grip strength. They also concluded that the best candidates for PRC are patients older than 35 years with an intact lunate facet of the distal radius and an intact capitate head. Richou and colleagues[49] reported long-term outcomes of PRC, with an average 9.6-year follow-up, in which 83% of patients were satisfied with their outcomes. Pain improved in all patients, grip strength was 76% of the contralateral side, total arc of flexion-extension was 76°, and average DASH scores were 31. Despite favorable clinical results, advancing radiographic staging was seen in 52% of patients.

Hohendorff and colleagues[50] recently published 1-year outcomes from an ongoing study, which compares 8 patients with STT fusion versus 11 patients with a PRC for stage IIIB Kienböck disease. These investigators reported slightly improved outcomes for the PRC group in terms of DASH scores, Mayo wrist scores, grip strength, and motion.

Crog and Stern[51] reported 10-year follow-up data on 21 patients treated with PRC, in whom 3 patients required radiocapitate arthrodesis. Even although 2 of those 3 patients had stage IV disease, they concluded that although it is a reliable procedure, PRC must be performed with caution

in patients with advanced stage disease. Likewise, DiDonna and colleagues[52] reported similar findings with PRC, cautioning against this procedure in patients younger than 35 years.

In an attempt to address capitoradial arthritis, Salomon and Eaton[53] also recommended an interpositional arthroplasty of the dorsal wrist capsule as an adjunct to PRC for patients with evidence of capitate head degenerative changes. In their study of 12 patients, with an average of 55 months of follow-up, 4 patients were treated with the addition of a dorsal capsule interpositional arthroplasty. There was a significant increase in postoperative flexion and grip strength, and most patients reported no pain.[53] An example of a patient with stage IIIB disease treated successfully with PRC can be seen in **Fig. 3**.

STT or SC arthrodesis

The goal of intercarpal arthrodesis (either the STT or SC joint) is to correct the flexed and rotated scaphoid in an attempt to stabilize the midcarpal joint, prevent further collapse, and halt degenerative change. Although several studies have reported good results for STT or SC arthrodesis in stage IIIB disease,[11,54,55] the results are not always satisfactory. Watson and colleagues[56] reported results of 28 patients treated with STT fusion, with an average of 51-month follow-up, and found that 78% of patients had good to excellent pain relief as well as improved grip strength and motion. These investigators advocated for fusion of the

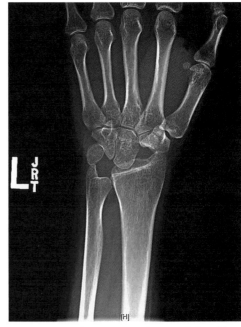

Fig. 3. Stage IIIB disease treated successfully with PRC.

scaphoid at 55° to 60° of flexion. Van den Dungen and colleagues[57] reported results of patients treated with either STT arthrodesis or conservative care. In this series, with a mean follow-up of 13 years, the STT arthrodesis group reported progressive pain, decreased motion, and longer rehabilitation time. Likewise, Tambe and colleagues[58] compared radiocarpal arthrodesis with intercarpal arthrodesis and reported more favorable outcomes in the radiocarpal arthrodesis group.

SC arthrodesis is another option for stage IIIB disease. Fusion of the SC joint has larger bony surfaces to fuse and only 1 articulation, compared with the STT fusion, with 3 separate articulations. Although reliable pain relief generally occurs with SC fusion, patients often have less midcarpal motion (eg, the dart thrower motion) when compared with STT fusion.[59,60]

Comparing STT fusion versus PRC has found similar outcomes between the 2 groups,[61] with no statistical difference with pain, grip strength, or range of motion.[62]

Grafting, arthroplasty, interposition

Other treatment options have been reported in an attempt to increase patient outcomes and satisfaction rates, decrease pain, and maintain motion and strength. In conjunction with an arthrodesis procedure, lunate excision with interposition or prosthetic grafting has been advocated as a pain-relieving procedure. Although initial results were favorable, silicone implants are no longer recommended as an option after lunate excision because of predictable synovitis and degeneration.[11,63,64] Zelouf and Ruby[65] have described a method of lunate bone grafting in conjunction with external fixation and reported improved grip strength, range of motion, and 80% pain relief.

As an alternative to bone grafting, Carroll[66] reported pain relief and improved motion in 10 patients, with 10-year follow-up for fascial interposition procedure after lunate excision. Furthermore, no patients had continued carpal collapse. Likewise, Ueba and colleagues[67] reported good to excellent results in 15 patients treated with palmaris longus/plantaris tendon interposition and distraction plating. All patients reported pain relief, grip strength was 90.2% of the contralateral wrist, range of motion increased by an average of 14.2°, and no significant carpal collapse occurred. Yajima and colleagues[68] supported this technique, with favorable pain reduction, improved motion, and improved grip strength in 12 patients with stage IIIB and 9 patients with stage IV treated with tendon roll arthroplasty and intercarpal pin fixation of either the STT or SC joint. Mariconda and colleagues confirmed clinically successful outcomes of 26

patients with an average of 125-month follow-up. Despite MRI advancement of disease in most patients, the average DASH scores were 7.7 and the mean visual analogue scale (VAS) score was 1.[69] As an alternative to silicone or tendon-ball interposition, Naum and colleagues[70] presented data on 16 patients undergoing titanium implantation after lunate excision and reported favorable outcomes in terms of grip strength, motion, and prevention of carpal collapse. Intercarpal fusions were performed in 7 of the 16 patients, but the stage of disease was not reported.

To our knowledge, there are no long-term studies, but novel techniques for tendon interposition are being described. Shigematsu and colleagues[71] reported favorable results using a rabbit model with various interposition techniques and found that a hybrid tendon roll using a tissue-engineering technique was capable of forming new bone and cartilage after transplantation into the lunate fossa.

Stage IV Disease

Stage IV disease shows similar radiographic findings as stage IIIB disease, with the addition of midcarpal and radiocarpal degenerative changes. Interventions to restore the lunate height or unload and revascularize the lunate have limited outcomes because of the degenerative changes that have occurred and the possibility of continued pain postoperatively. Thus, salvage procedures are often performed in patients who present with stage IV Kienböck disease. The mainstays of treatment of stage IV disease include PRC, wrist arthrodesis, wrist denervation, or wrist arthroplasty.

PRC is an option for stage IV Kienböck disease, but is cautioned against if there is significant degenerative change of the capitate head. As mentioned earlier, interposition arthroplasty of the distal radius with the dorsal wrist capsule combined with PRC can be useful if mild degenerative changes are present within the capitate.[53] El-Mowafi and colleagues[72] reviewed 12 patients with stage IV Kienböck disease treated with PRC, with an average 2-year follow-up. There was 1 failure, which required fusion, but 9 of 12 patients had complete pain relief, associated with a 70° flexion-extension arc and maintenance of 80% grip strength compared with the contralateral side. Contrary to this finding, Croog and Stern[51] reported favorable results with PRC for stage IIIB disease, but poor outcomes associated with radiocapitate degeneration in patients with stage IV disease. Thus, although PRC is a motion-sparing option for stage IV disease, careful patient selection is warranted.

Wrist denervation reduces pain, but questions exist as to the extent of functional outcomes, the correct method of denervation, and whether it has any advantage long-term compared with PRC or wrist arthrodesis. Buck-Gramcko[73] reported 76% to 88% patient satisfaction after wrist denervation, either in conjunction with another procedure or alone, for the treatment of Kienböck disease. Despite radiographic progression of continued degeneration, favorable outcomes in terms of pain control have been reported.[74] In the senior author's experience, wrist denervation works for centrally located pain and provides a temporary midterm motion-sparing solution.

Wrist arthroplasty provides a motion salvage procedure replacing the damaged proximal carpal row and distal radius articular surface. Proper patient selection is paramount, given activity restrictions that accompany wrist arthroplasty postoperatively. In 2012, Nydick and colleagues[75] reported on 23 arthroplasties in 22 patients for a combination of Kienböck, osteoarthritis, and rheumatoid arthritis followed for 28 months. VAS pain scores improved from 8 to 2.2, total arc of flexion/extension averaged 90°, and there was no evidence of prosthetic loosening. Complications occurred in 7, and 1 patient required revision surgery. Other studies report a higher incidence of complications. In a questionnaire sent to 38 patients after wrist arthroplasty, 37 patients reported improved pain relief, despite there being 4 dislocations and 1 case of complex regional pain syndrome.[76] Hemiarthroplasty, combining resurfacing of the distal radius and PRC, is a new and evolving modality. There are no medium-term or long-term outcome studies validating its usage, but case reports are suggestive of short-term success.[77,78]

Wrist arthrodesis is a motion-saving salvage procedure when other treatment modalities have failed, or when degeneration has progressed to a state at which other treatments are no longer considered. Arthrodesis removes all motion within the volar to dorsal flexion/extension arc, but maintains pronation and supination.

Salvage procedures for stage IV disease should address the degree of degenerative change and provide adequate function and pain relief. However, questions about the ideal treatment option for advanced Kienböck disease still remain, and patient expectations must be discussed and considered before procedural selection.

SUMMARY

Kienböck disease is defined by AVN of the lunate, with a predictable pattern of lunate collapse, carpal change, and degeneration, resulting from an apparent combination of vascular, anatomic, and traumatic insults. Advancements are still being made with regards to the cause, pathophysiology, and preferred method of treatment of each of the various stages of Kienböck disease. Although the goals of pain relief, motion preservation, strength maintenance, and function outcomes are paramount to success, there is no 1 procedure that consistently and reliably achieves these outcomes. Thus, with further advancements in treatment and results of long-term outcome studies, answers should be obtained to some of these still unresolved topics.

REFERENCES

1. Peste JL. Discussion. Bull Soc Anat Paris 1843;18:169.
2. [translated] Kienböck R, Peltier L. Concerning traumatic malacia of the lunate and its consequences: degeneration and compression fractures [reprint]. Clin Orthop Relat Res 1980;(149):4–8.
3. Hulten O. Uber anatomische Variationen der Handgelenkknochen. Acta Radiol 1928;9:155–68 [in German].
4. Gelberman RH, Bauman TD, Menon J, et al. The vascularity of the lunate bone and Kienböck's disease. J Hand Surg Am 1980;5:272–8.
5. Antuna Zapico JM. Malacia del Semilunar. Tesis doctora, Industrias y Editorial Sever Cuesta. Valladolid (España): Universidad de Valladolid; 1966 [in Spanish].
6. D'Horre K, DeSmet L, Verellen K, et al. Negative ulnar variance is not a risk factor for Kienböck's Disease. J Hand Surg Am 1994;19:229–31.
7. Nakamura R, Imaeda T, Miura T. Radial shortening for Kienböck's disease: factors affecting the operative result. J Hand Surg Br 1990;15:40–5.
8. Tsuge S, Nakamura R. Anatomical risk factors for Kienböck's disease. J Hand Surg Br 1993;18:70–5.
9. Wantanabe K, Nakamura R, Horii E, et al. Biomechanical analysis of radial wedge osteotomy for the treatment of Kienböck's disease. J Hand Surg Am 1993;18:686–90.
10. Panagis JS, Gelberman RH, Taleisnik J, et al. The arterial anatomy of the human carpus. Part II: the intraosseous vascularity. J Hand Surg Am 1983;8:375–82.
11. Lichtman DM, Mack GR, MacDonald RI, et al. Kienböck's disease: the role of silicone replacement arthroplasty. J Bone Joint Surg Am 1977;59:899–908.
12. Culp RW, Schaffer J, Osterman AL, et al. Kienböck's disease in a patient with Crohn's enteritis treated with corticosteroids. J Hand Surg Am 1989;14:294–6.
13. Allan CH, Joshi A, Lichtman DM. Kienböck's disease: diagnosis and treatment. J Am Acad Orthop Surg 2001;9:128–36.

14. Luo J, Diao E. Kienböck's disease: an approach to treatment. Hand Clin 2006;22:465–73.

15. Schiond F, Eslami S, Ledoux P. Kienböck's disease. J Bone Joint Surg Br 2008;90:133–9.

16. Schiltenwolf M, Martini AK, Mau HC, et al. Further investigations of the intraosseous pressure characteristics in necrotic lunates. J Hand Surg Am 1996; 21:754–8.

17. Divebliss B, Baratz M. Kienböck disease. J Am Soc Surg Hand 2001;1:61–72.

18. Takami H, Takahashi S, Ando M, et al. Open reduction of chronic lunate and perilunate dislocations. Arch Orthop Trauma Surg 1996;115:104–7.

19. Beckenbaugh RD, Shives TC, Dobyns JH, et al. Kienböck's disease: the natural history of Kienböck's disease and consideration of lunate fractures. Clin Orthop 1980;149:98–106.

20. Hashizume H, Asahara H, Nishida K, et al. Histopathology of Kienböck's disease: correlation with magnetic resonance imaging and other imaging techniques. J Hand Surg Br 1996;21:89–93.

21. Quezner DE, Linscheid RL, Vidal MA, et al. Trispiral tomographic staging of Kienböck's disease. J Hand Surg Am 1997;22:396–403.

22. Stahl F. On lunatomalacia (Kienböck's disease): a clinical and roentgenological study, especially on its pathogenesis and the late results of immobilization treatment. Acta Chir Scand 1947;(126):3.

23. Wolfe SW. Kienböck's disease. Green's operative hand surgery. 6th edition. philadelphia: Elsevier; 2011.

24. Tajima T. An investigation of the treatment of Kienböck's disease. J Bone Joint Surg Am 1966;48: 1649.

25. Taniguchi T, Tamaki T, Nakatan N. Long-term results of non-surgical treatment in Kienböck's disease. J Jpn Soc Surg Hand 1993;9:962–8.

26. Kristensen SS, Thomassen E, Christensen F. Ulnar variance in Kienböck's disease. J Hand Surg Br 1986;11:258.

27. Delaere O, Dury M, Molderez A, et al. Conservative versus operative treatment for Kienböck's disease. J Hand Surg Br 1998;23:33–6.

28. Keith PP, Nuttall D, Trail I. Long-term outcome of nonsurgically managed Kienböck's disease. J Hand Surg Am 2004;29:63–7.

29. Horii E, Garcia-Elias M, Bishop AT, et al. Effect on force transmission across the carpus in procedures used to treat Kienböck's disease. J Hand Surg Am 1990;15:393–400.

30. Trumble T, Glisson RR, Seaber AV, et al. A biomechanical comparison of the methods for treating Kienböck's disease. J Hand Surg Am 1986;11:88–93.

31. Nakamura R, Horii E, Imaeda T. Excessive radial shortening in Kienböck's disease. J Hand Surg Br 1990;15:46–8.

32. Quenzer DE, Dobyns JH, Linscheid RL, et al. Radial recession osteotomy for Kienböck's disease. J Hand Surg Am 1997;22:386–95.

33. Watanabe T, Takahara M, Tsuchida H, et al. Long-term follow-up of radial shortening osteotomy for Kienböck disease. J Bone Joint Surg Am 2008; 90:1705–11.

34. Raven EE, Haverkamp D, Marti RK. Outcome of Kienböck's disease 22 years after distal radius shortening osteotomy. Clin Orthop Relat Res 2007;460:137–41.

35. Linscheid RL. Ulnar lengthening and shortening. Hand Clin 1987;3:69–79.

36. Sheetz KK, Bishop AT, Berger RA. The arterial blood supply of the distal radius and ulna and its potential use in vascularized pedicled bone grafts. J Hand Surg Am 1995;20:902–14.

37. Bochud RC, Buchler U. Kienböck's disease, early stage 3: height reconstruction and core revascularization of the lunate. J Hand Surg Br 1994;19: 466–78.

38. Tamai S, Yajima H, Ono H. Revascularization procedures in the treatment of Kienböck's disease. Hand Clin 1993;9:455–66.

39. Hori Y, Tamai S, Okuda H, et al. Blood vessel transplantation to bone. J Hand Surg Am 1979; 4:23–33.

40. Moran SL, Cooney WP, Berger RA, et al. The use of the 4 + 5 extensor compartmental vascularized bone graft for the treatment of Kienböck's disease. J Hand Surg Am 2005;30:50–8.

41. Moran SL, Cooney WP, Berger RA, et al. Vascularized bone grafts for the treatment of Kienböck's disease: ten year experience. Presented at American Society for Surgery of the Hand. Phoenix, October 4th, 2002.

42. Almquist EE. Capitate shortening in the treatment of Kienböck's disease. Hand Clin 1993;9: 505–12.

43. Viola RW, Kiser PK, Bach AW. Biomechanical analysis of capitate shortening with capitate hamate fusion in the treatment of Kienböck's disease. J Hand Surg Am 1998;23:395–401.

44. Beredjiklian P. Kienböck 's disease. J Hand Surg Am 2009;34:167–75.

45. Koh S, Nakamura R, Horii E, et al. Surgical outcome of radial osteotomy for Kienböck's disease–minimum 10 years of follow-up. J Hand Surg Am 2003;28:910–6.

46. Takahara M, Watanabe T, Tsuchida H, et al. Long-term follow-up of radial shortening osteotomy for Kienböck disease: surgical technique. J Bone Joint Surg Am 2009;91(Suppl 2):184–90.

47. Illarramendi AA, Schulz C, De Carli P. The surgical treatment of Kienböck's disease by radius and ulna metaphyseal core decompression. J Hand Surg Am 2001;26:252–60.

48. Wall LB, Stern PJ. Proximal row carpectomy. Hand Clin 2013;29:69–78.

49. Richou J, Chuinard C, Moineau G, et al. Proximal row carpectomy: long term results. Chir Main 2010;29:10–5.

50. Hohendorff B, Muhldorfer-Fodor M, Kalb K. STT arthrodesis versus proximal row carpectomy for Lichtman stage IIIB Kienböck's disease: first results of an ongoing observational study. Arch Orthop Trauma Surg 2012;132:1327–34.

51. Croog AS, Stern PJ. Proximal row carpectomy for advanced Kienböck's disease: average 10-year follow-up. J Hand Surg Am 2008;33:1122–30.

52. DiDonna ML, Kiefhaber TR, Stern PJ. Proximal row carpectomy: study with a minimum of ten years of follow-up. J Bone Joint Surg Am 2004;86:2359–65.

53. Salomon GD, Eaton RG. Proximal row carpectomy with partial capitate resection. J Hand Surg Am 1996;12:2–8.

54. Iwasaki N, Genda E, Barrance PJ, et al. Biomechanical analysis of limited intercarpal fusion for the treatment of Kienböck's disease: a three-dimensional theoretical study. J Orthop Res 1998; 16:256–63.

55. Linscheid RL. Kienböck's disease. Instr Course Lect 1992;41:45–53.

56. Watson HK, Monacelli DM, Milford RS, et al. Treatment of Kienböck's disease with scaphotrazio-trapezoid arthrodesis. J Hand Surg Am 1996;21:9–15.

57. Van den Dungen S, Dury M, Foucher G, et al. Conservative treatment versus scaphotrapeziotrapezoid arthrodesis for Kienböck's disease. A retrospective study. Chir Main 2006;25:141–5.

58. Tambe AD, Trail IA, Stanley JK. Wrist fusion versus limited carpal fusion in advanced Kienböck's disease. Int Orthop 2005;29:355–8.

59. Pisano SM, Peimer CA, Wheeler DR. Scaphocapitate intercarpal arthrodesis. J Hand Surg Am 1991;16:328–33.

60. Sennwald GR, Ufenast H. Scaphocapitate arthrodesis for the treatment of Kienböck's disease. J Hand Surg Am 1995;20:506–10.

61. Condit DP, Idler RS, Fischer TJ, et al. Preoperative factors and outcome after lunate decompression for Kienböck's disease. J Hand Surg Am 1993;18:691–6.

62. Nakamura R, Horii E, Watanabe K. Proximal row carpectomy versus limited wrist arthrodesis for advanced Kienböck's disease. J Hand Surg Br 1998;23:741–5.

63. Alexander AH, Turner MA, Alexander CE, et al. Lunate silicone replacement arthroplasty for Kienböck's disease: a long-term follow-up. J Hand Surg Am 1990;15:401–7.

64. Kato H, Usui M, Minami A. Long-term results of Kienböck's disease treated by excisional arthroplasty with a silicone implant or coiled palmaris longus tendon. J Hand Surg Am 1986;11:645–53.

65. Zelouf DS, Ruby LK. External fixation and cancellous bone grafting for Kienböck's disease: a preliminary report. J Hand Surg Am 1996;21:746–53.

66. Carroll RE. Long term review of fascial replacement after excision of the carpal lunate bone. Clin Orthop Relat Res 1997;342:59–63.

67. Ueba Y, Nosaka K, Seto Y, et al. An operative procedure for advanced Kienböck's disease. Excision of the lunate and subsequent replacement with a tendon-ball implant. J Orthop Sci 1999;4:207–15.

68. Yajima H, Kobata Y, Yamauchi T, et al. Advanced Kienböck's disease treated with implantation of a tendon roll and temporary partial fixation of the wrist. Scand J Plast Reconstr Surg Hand Surg 2004;38:340–6.

69. Mariconda M, Soscia E, Sirignano C, et al. Long-term clinical results and MRI changes after tendon ball arthroplasty for advanced Kienböck's disease. J Hand Surg Eur Vol 2013;38(5):508–14.

70. Naum SC, VanGorp CC, DeHeer DH, et al. Titanium lunate implant arthroplasty for Kienböck's disease: one to nine year follow-up. Presented at American Society for Surgery of the Hand. Denver, September 11, 1997.

71. Shigematsu K, Hattori K, Kobata YM, et al. Treatment of Kienböck's disease with cultured stem cell-seeded hybrid tendon roll interposition arthroplasty: experimental study. J Orthop Sci 2006;11: 198–203.

72. El-Mowafi H, El-Hadidi M, El-Karef E. Proximal row carpectomy: a motion-preserving procedure in the treatment of advanced Kienböck's disease. Acta Orthop Belg 2006;72:530–4.

73. Buck-Gramcko D. Wrist denervation procedures in the treatment of Kienböck's disease. Hand Clin 1993;9:517–20.

74. Braga-Silva J, Romàn JA, Padoin AV. Wrist denervation for painful conditions of the wrist. J Hand Surg Am 2011;36:961–6.

75. Nydick JA, Greenberg SM, Stone JD, et al. Clinical outcomes of total wrist arthroplasty. J Hand Surg Am 2012;37:1580–4.

76. Strunk S, Bracker W. Wrist joint arthroplasty: results after 41 prostheses. Handchir Mikrochir Plast Chir 2009;41:141–7.

77. Boyer JS, Adams BD. Distal radius hemiarthroplasty combined with proximal row carpectomy: a case report. Iowa Orthop J 2010;30:168.

78. Culp RW. Distal radius hemiarthroplasty combined with proximal row carpectomy. Presented at 67th Annual Meeting of the American Society for Surgery of the Hand. Chicago, September 2012.

Index

Orthop Clin N Am 45 (2014) 153–156
http://dx.doi.org/10.1016/S0030-5898(13)00174-0
0030-5898/14/$ – see front matter © 2014 Elsevier Inc. All rights reserved.